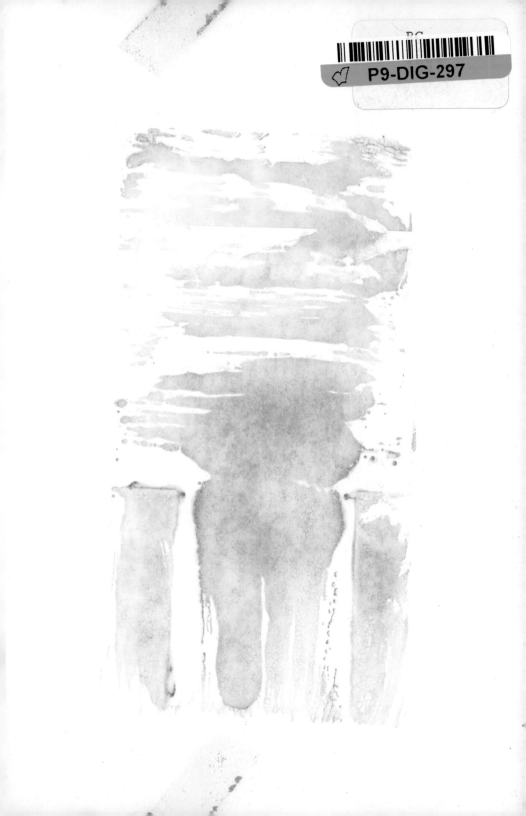

PORTRAIT OF APHASIA

David Knox

PORTRAIT OF APHASIA

Wayne State University Press
Detroit
1971

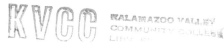

Published simultaneously in Canada
by The Copp Clark Publishing Company
517 Wellington Street, West
Toronto 2B, Canada.
Second printing, 1972
Library of Congress Catalog Card Number 76–146591
International Standard Book Number 0–8143–1439–2

To My Wife, Betty
who likes that name,
and preferred that her real name
not be used.

CONTENTS

Grateful acknowledgment is extended to Josephine Simonson for proposing that this book be written, and for lending helpful encouragement after it was started.

I am also indebted to my wife for generously permitting the details of her travail to be published. Thanks are due her also for the expert help she provided in proofreading.

INTRODUCTION

Aphasia is one of medicine's most dramatic phenomena. In simple terms it means the impairment or loss of the ability to use or understand written or spoken language. Actually it is a much more complex subject. It is due in most cases to acquired damage of the so-called "language area" located on the left side of the brain. This is usually caused by a "stroke" which cuts off the blood supply to this area but a brain tumor, head injury, and other less common noxious processes may have the same effect.

The protean manifestations of aphasia may vary from a mild or partial aphasia (dysphasia) in which the patient occasionally uses a wrong word to the patient with global aphasia who can neither utter nor understand a single syllable. In between lies a broad spectrum of dysphasias of varying complexity and severity. Aphasia is intimately related to apraxia, the inability to perform a simple movement or activity despite the absence of any paralysis; agnosia, the inability to speak the name of an object or person although speech is otherwise intact; and alexia, the in-

11

ability to read a word or even a single letter. Agraphia, acalculia, and ideational apraxia are other related neurological deficits. There are patients able to carry on normal conversations who, if asked to name an object such as a comb or watch, are unable to do so although they may demonstrate its use by pantomime. There are dysphasic patients who can name animate but not inanimate objects; others who can name the color of a red or green traffic light but cannot tell whether it means stop or go, yet others who can name eyeglasses if they are worn but not if they are held in the hand. An aphasic patient may be unable to speak a single word but when he is frightened or angered he may let fly with a stream of profanity.

Aphasia is closely related to the most remarkable of all biological phenomena, the human memory. The study of aphasia has greatly expanded our knowledge of the learning process and other intellectual mechanisms.

The problem of the nature of aphasia has challenged the curiosity and investigative abilities of neurologists, physiologists, anatomists, and even philosophers. Early in the nineteenth century, Lordat, a French physician and student of the nature of speech, himself suffered an attack of aphasia. After partial recovery, he wrote a treatise on his experiences but could not read aloud what he himself had written! Many of the great neurologists of the past hundred and fifty years have contributed to our knowledge of aphasia. Among them are Broca, Wernicke, Kussmaul, Jackson, Charcot, Head, Henschen, Goldstein, Wilson, Allen, Starr, Mills, Critchley, and Nielsen. Even Sigmund Freud, who was a neurologist before he became interested in psychoanalysis, wrote extensively on the subject and made major additions to our knowledge of aphasia. Many neurologists today consider these contributions his only truly scientific work.

The works of these men and others currently engaged in the problem is enormously interesting to the scientific investigator, but what of the aphasic patient, his family and friends, his physician and others who must work with him personally and professionally? There is probably no disability more frustrating to the patient than aphasia. The tears commonly shed by the aphasic patient are those of frustration. H. L. Mencken, a master of language and author of books on language, was never able to speak again after suffering a stroke. How does the patient react to this ultimate frustration? Is there a road back? The answer for some is yes; for others, partly; for others, no.

In *Portrait of Aphasia,* Mr. David Knox describes his wife Betty's attack of aphasia and the struggle and drama of their attempt to deal with it. It is an odyssey of two very remarkable people.

Mr. Knox writes with great clarity and readability on a subject difficult for a specialist in the field, much less a layman. Mr. Knox accomplishes a most formidable task, conveying in understandable fashion many of the difficulties the aphasic patient has with language. He gives at times an almost subjective view of the aphasic, a position which the afflicted person cannot himself convey because of the nature of his language deficit. This alone is a remarkable achievement. It is probably an actual advantage that the author does not possess technical expertise in the field allowing him thereby to better communicate this material to the general reader.

An important aspect of this story is that the patient does not fully recover from the aphasia. This is true of most aphasics in whom loss of speech has persisted for more than a few days. Mrs. Knox has moderately severe residuals and it is this type of patient who needs most to be understood in the social and professional contacts of all of us. Such an account has more substance and meaning than the story of an aphasic patient who recovers completely or nearly so. Mr. Knox's own emotional responses to the situations of encouragement and discouragement are genuine, the real thing.

The general reader will find *Portrait of Aphasia* an absorbing and exciting story. It will give great rewards to the family and friends of aphasic patients and to those working in the field of aphasia, namely speech therapists, physicians, nurses, and those in the field of physical rehabilitation. Woven into the story are many useful and important suggestions for helping the aphasic patient to relearn language.

Reading *Portrait of Aphasia* was a great pleasure to me as a neurologist both because of my professional interest and its literary and human appeal.

Joseph L. Whelan, M.D.

1

Lightning Strikes

The shattering episode cast no warning shadow. The tropical sun poured through the parted drapes, drenching the bed and proclaiming one more in a sequence of brilliant Mexican days. My mind, still drowsy, savored the tranquillity of our carefree holiday at Las Brisas as I momentarily suppressed the urging of wakefulness. Acapulco in March was all that we had expected. Leisurely continental breakfasts on the patio; swimming in our private fresh-water pool, or in the briny beach pool; sightseeing in the pink jeep that earmarks Las Brisas; cocktails on the patio with neighbors; and pleasureful dining at a different exotic restaurant each evening to the accompaniment of strolling *mariachis*— thus had we pleasantly recharged our run-down batteries.

And contemplating the future was satisfying. I brushed aside the intervening days of necessary work and focused on the anticipated enjoyment of visits to other exotic places of perpetual sunshine. With the children now grown and retirement only four years away, there would be much more opportunity to travel.

Languorously my mind caressed the expanding future, until I was brought up short by the urgency of the present. We had to get moving; our plane was to leave for Mexico City at one o'clock and we were only half-packed.

Though I noticed that Betty was not stirring it did not occur to me that anything might be wrong. On vacations she often waited for me to start the day by a word of endearment or a brief kiss. But this time there was no response—no answer to my "good morning." Just those two big brown eyes staring at me. As I took her in my arms I told her to quit play acting, we had work to do and must get moving. Still no answer. Slowly, oh so slowly, I became aware that something was wrong. Fear and then panic seized me. I frantically tried to get her to respond, to show some sign of awareness. What had happened to her? What should I do? Had she suddenly lost her mind—or was it amnesia? I had never before been confronted with anything like this and I was almost paralyzed with fear—yet I knew that I had to do something.

I told her I would get a doctor and I sensed that she understood, for she offered no objection. When I reached a phone I somehow made the desk clerk realize that my need was urgent. A half-hour later the house doctor appeared, and after a very brief examination indicated, in broken English, that this case was beyond his ability to help. He obviously had had more experience with the treatment of hangovers and intestinal upsets so common among tourists. But he promised he would call a capable physician in Acapulco, which was some distance from Las Brisas. I was impelled to ask him to hurry, even though I knew that it would have no

16

effect on the outcome. Rarely does anything happen quickly in Mexico.

After about a half-hour a note was delivered to me at our cottage. The note was written in longhand on the reverse side of a Las Brisas Hilton reservation form, and read as follows:

Mr. Knox
   I contact Dr. Mendoza. He will be able to come to see your wife in about 1 or 1½ hours, in the mean time keep her quiet and try that she sleep and rest. Don't move her.
                                            Dr. Zuloaga

While I waited, a hundred questions flashed through my mind in almost uninterrupted sequence. Would we be able to use our plane reservations? Since she was obviously very ill, should I telephone my family in Michigan? How good was the hospital in Acapulco? Would language be a problem? Where could I find living quarters for myself during a prolonged stay in a vacation city? Should I consult with my home physician by telephone? What caused this thing to happen to her, whatever it might be? Could I have done anything to prevent it? And so, on and on, went the questions.

After what seemed an eternity, and two more nervous walks down the hill to the telephone, Dr. Mendoza finally arrived about 10:30 A.M. My confidence in his medical proficiency, admittedly low at first, rose considerably when he unpacked his portable EKG apparatus and proceeded to make the connections preparatory to a heart examination.

After pronouncing that Betty's heart was acting normally, he proceeded with tests of reflexes, and requested her to perform certain limb and finger movements including walking. I was encouraged that she seemed to be trying to respond to his questions, but the nature of some of her responses was baffling. She would invariably raise her left hand when asked to raise her right one, and seemed quite confused. She uttered no words but was able to stand and walk, with some help from me, and improved with each attempt. I was to become much more familiar with these neurological tests as time went on; but at this point the procedure had little meaning for me except as medical hodge-podge leading to the all-important final diagnosis. It was not long in coming.

"Your wife has had a stroke," said Dr. Mendoza. "She has some paralysis, limited to her left hand, but no immobilizing paralysis at this time. However, her speech is definitely damaged and she should be hospitalized as soon as possible."

Then I put to him the question uppermost in my mind. "We have reservations on Aeronaves for Mexico City at one o'clock, and on Canadian Pacific Airlines to Detroit tomorrow morning. Can she take this trip? Can I get her home to a hospital?" After contemplating this briefly he said, "Yes, she could be considered ambulatory under the circumstances." I was so relieved to hear this that I did not even shudder when he said the bill would be 500 pesos, and I proceeded to sign over to him two $20 traveler's checks, forgetting to ask for a receipt. He made out a prescription for anticoagulant pills to be given to her, one every six hours, and went on his way, leaving me with my patient.

In retrospect, the return trip seems like a nightmare of frustrations. The long wait for filling the prescription was minor compared to the delay at Acapulco Airport,

18

which had no air-cooling system. I had Betty seated in the waiting room for as long as possible, but we joined the line at the exit gate as soon as it formed to be sure of getting seats together. We did succeed in getting adjoining seats, but what a price we paid in discomfort and fatigue! I felt so sorry for Betty, standing there in the humid heat for so long, but she was to repeat this display of fortitude many times in the future.

We arrived at the hotel in Mexico City without incident, and Betty went to bed immediately while I ordered some light nourishment for her. She ate sparingly, and since it was time for the second anticoagulant pill, I gave it to her. Within a few minutes her stomach rejected the pill along with the little food she had eaten. I decided then not to give her any more of the pills until she had been examined by our regular physician. Later I learned that the general use of anticoagulants immediately following a stroke is considered by some medical people to be controversial. It has been suggested that in some particular cases of stroke the thinning of the blood would tend to spread the damage to a larger area of the brain. Yet there are many fine medical people, I am told, who confidently prescribe anticoagulants following strokes. That I made the correct decision in withholding the anticoagulant pill is questionable.

Although I rested in bed that night, sleep was not permitted to soothe my troubled mind. I was like the animal in the forest, semiaware, with ears cocked to intercept the slightest unusual sound. After arousing Betty the next morning I was pleasantly surprised to find that she needed a minimum of help in dressing and applying her usual cosmetics. She was very much aware of her appearance and needed help only in locating the items that she used.

Our tourist guide in Mexico City met us at the hotel as scheduled and escorted us to the airport. Earlier I had telephoned Betty's sister in Detroit and asked her to make the necessary arrangements for Betty to enter Beaumont Hospital that evening, and to notify other members of our family. Confidently I approached the Canadian Pacific Airways desk to check in with our tickets, thankful that I had reservations as I listened to people ahead of me clamoring and pleading for seats.

I was totally unprepared for what followed, and I became quite belligerent when the clerk said he could not give me seats on this plane because my tickets had not been reconfirmed twenty-four hours in advance. My disturbed mental condition would not admit any responsibility on my part for this terrible turn of events; I berated my Mexican guide for not reconfirming, and I berated the airline, to no avail. The clerk was adamant even after I had calmed down and told him of my wife's illness and her need for hospitalization.

Helpless, and in desperation approaching tears, I asked the guide what we could do. He should have been much more familiar than I with this kind of problem, but he was of little help until I suggested we see the manager of the airline. My guide was able to locate a person of higher authority in an obscure office to the rear of the ticket counter. After I described my predicament to this person and showed him the prescription signed by Dr. Mendoza as verification of the illness, he took my ticket and disappeared. After some period of waiting I realized that I was sitting there without a ticket and I had no identification of the man who had taken it. My ineffectual tourist guide had left me some time before, and Betty was sitting alone out in the crowded waiting room.

Sweating it out in this back room, I tried as best I could to be optimistic about the outcome. They couldn't possibly deny the flight reservations I had made and paid for two months earlier. Someone had to find a way to put us on this flight.

Yet I found myself returning again and again to the dark probability that we would have to remain in Mexico City a few days or possibly a week longer. What would I do with Betty? I decided that the answer to that question would best be given by a capable physician. But how would I locate a capable physician? I concerned myself with as many of the potential problems as I could while sitting and waiting. I wanted to go out to Betty and reassure her that she was not forgotten or abandoned, but I was afraid that the man with my tickets might return at any moment.

After what seemed to be an interminable period of waiting, the airline officer returned and proceeded to write on a slip of paper.

"Are you going to put us on this flight?" I pleaded.

Slowly his whispered answer came in the affirmative. "But I want you to wait back here out of sight until I call you," he said. "Too many people are out there in front demanding and expecting to get on this flight, and I want you to stay here where you can't be seen until I tell you the flight is ready."

I shall be eternally grateful for what this stranger did for us once he understood our predicament. He was only the first of many who showed the great depth of human kindness and understanding, extending a helping hand when it was most needed.

And what part did the anticoagulant prescription, signed by a Mexican doctor, play in this fortunate sequence? Though the written prescription may have been controversial, it certainly served a useful purpose by helping to convince the airline officer that I was telling the truth and not employing trickery.

We were the last to board the aircraft and I was so thankful to be homeward bound that the separation of our seats did not seem of great importance. Betty was only three rows away and I was able to help her with the eating tools when dinner was served. She appeared confused in the use of her knife and fork, a confusion which would persist for several weeks.

It was heartwarming to have so many of our family waiting for us when we arrived home. Betty immediately assumed the role of hostess, although silent, and concerned herself that everyone had a place to sit. By pantomime she even urged them to have refreshments. This exhibition was reassuring; she was able to recognize people and her personality was basically unchanged. Of course, everyone insisted they were more concerned with her sitting and resting after the long trip from Mexico. Within an hour my son had driven us to Beaumont Hospital where she was admitted as a patient.

Following a preliminary examination the next morning our physician confirmed the diagnosis made by Dr. Mendoza in Mexico: Betty had suffered a stroke. He proceeded to describe the cerebral vascular accident (CVA) in layman's terms, and I understood for the first time how the speech areas of her brain had been damaged. The regions of speech initiation and word understanding were no longer functioning normally. The vocal chords were undamaged and would respond normally if the brain could generate and transmit the proper impulse. But without the impulse from the brain there is no speech. The extent of the brain damage varies from patient to patient, and in Betty's case would have to be determined by a series of neurological tests during her hospitalization. He then delivered the crushing news that even with therapy it would take as long as a year to recover speech ability, and possibly longer.

It is difficult for me to believe now that I was so lacking in knowledge about the relationship of stroke to speech. It took all the fortitude I could muster at that moment to absorb the impact of what was ahead of us. Our church pastor was with me during the doctor's discourse and gave me encouragement that I would have the strength and spiritual stamina to make the necessary adjustments. His consoling contention proved to be correct. Fortunately it was not possible at this point to bring the blurred future into sharp focus, or to foresee any new and unexpected events. A future fraught with obstacles that are not clearly defined can generate the strength necessary to overcome them. Complete clarity often tips the scales in favor of futility.

Although I returned to my job the following day, a bout with the flu and dysentery laid me low for a few days. A daughter is indeed a comfort in such a situation. Janet not only cared for me, but made daily visits to her mother at the hospital. It warms my heart that Betty still saves and cherishes a letter I wrote to her during this period, explaining and minimizing my illness, and affirming my love and concern for her. I could not tell at that time how much she understood of what was written. It is now obvious, from the fact of her saving the letter, that she understood more than I realized. And if the letter was not completely understood, certainly there is evidence that she was aware of the intent and feeling of the message, and its importance to her morale.

During Betty's two weeks in the hospital, extensive neurological tests were conducted which were not particularly disturbing to the patient but which provided more information about the damage to the brain. In addition, however, there were two neurosurgical procedures conducted which were of far more concern to me. These were very severe on the patient and they required a high degree of surgical skill.

The first was the pneumoencephalogram, and consisted of injecting air into the lower back region. For this test, the patient is sitting in an upright position. The air, being lighter than body fluids, rises and displaces the liquid which surrounds the brain tissue and insulates it from the hard bone of the skull. The air provides a low density space between the brain and the skull bone to permit taking pictures with X-rays which reveal the external outline of the brain. No general anesthetic is used because the patient is required to sit upright. The period of recovery is probably the worst phase of this procedure, for the patient must lie quietly in bed with a minimum of movement for a period of twenty-four hours and experience an excruciating headache, particularly when the head is moved, while the air is absorbed into the system.

The second procedure was called an arteriogram. It

involves producing a series of pictures of the skull which will reveal the blood-circulating system in the brain after a suitable dye material is injected into the blood stream. The dye material is opaque to the X-ray used for pictures, and serves to reveal a number of possible malfunctions in the brain arteries, as well as the location of the malfunction, that would explain the present condition of the patient. The knowledge gained from these procedures is useful in evaluating the cause and extent of the damage, and in determining the future treatment and activity of the patient.

To my knowledge none of these tests positively revealed the specific cause of the brain damage. No evidence of a tumor was found but the tests indirectly revealed that a small blood clot, not precisely located, was the probable cause of the damage, shutting off the flow of nurturing lifeblood to the affected area. Perhaps the greatest benefit of these tests was a negative sort of knowledge that there was no evidence of tumor, either benign or malignant. As soon as the medical specialists had submitted their findings to our doctor, an internist, he recommended that I arrange to have Betty start speech therapy as soon as possible after she was discharged from the hospital. He strongly emphasized doing this immediately, for it has been found that postponing therapy makes recovery slower and less complete.

Apologetically, he said there was no accredited speech therapist associated with William Beaumont Hospital or with any other hospital in the northern suburban area of Detroit. But he highly recommended a woman therapist associated with Henry Ford Hospital in Detroit and suggested that I call her.

It was during this hospitalization period that I plunged into planning for the days ahead, planning that would allow me to carry out my duties and responsibilities directing the industrial engineering activity of a multiplant metal-working company, and at the same time provide for a speech therapy program for my wife. It was mandatory that I continue working if I was to bear the added financial burden of the speech therapy program. Since my position carried considerable responsibility I knew I must devote most of my time and energy to being a reasonably successful engineer. It was immediately obvious that I would need a capable housekeeper.

I soon found out that finding a suitable housekeeper would not be easy; only as a last resort would I consider asking our youngest daughter to interrupt her college education with only a little over a year left to graduation. I realized that the woman would have to be acceptable to Betty if she were to make rapid progress in therapy. I wanted to free Betty from the problems and responsibilities of the home as much as possible and provide a restful atmosphere in which she could feel comfortable. But how to find such a person?

The answer, of course, lies in talking to as many people as possible about the problem. It is amazing how rapidly and widespread such information can be transmitted by the personal conversation chain.

Berniece came to us through a sister of a mutual friend of Betty and her sister. This sounds a bit complicated but that's the way such information gets around. Betty's sister gave us a description of Berniece as a widow, not young, who had been caring for an elderly man until his recent death. Berniece was highly recom-

mended as a competent and honest person and was seeking another position as a housekeeper.

I brought Betty home from the hospital on a Saturday, two weeks after her stroke in Mexico, and Berniece came for an interview Sunday afternoon. In such a situation she was interviewing us as much as we were interviewing her. This would be her home for an indefinite period—as it turned out, for nearly three years—and certainly she was interested in knowing what kind of people we were, what her living quarters would be like, what facilities were provided for keeping house, and whether she felt comfortable with us.

We, in turn, needed to know something of her background and, most importantly, how Betty would react to her personally. A feeling for these things usually can be derived from drawing a person into conversation, starting with subjects of common interest and leading into questions that cannot be answered with a simple yes or no.

It did not take us long to agree that Berniece would come to live with us the following Tuesday, with the privilege of going to her daughter's home, about twenty miles away, every Sunday to be with her family and to attend the church where she liked to worship. It so happened that Berniece's religious faith and denomination coincided with ours and I felt at the time that this was a desirable factor. In retrospect I still feel that the aphasic patient should be confronted with a very minimum of frictional circumstances, and a religious difference could be a minor irritant.

27

2

Speech Therapy—Phase 1

In a sense, language therapy started almost immediately after Betty's discharge from the hospital, but it concerned writing rather than speaking. Ironically, I had provided for several hundred dollars' worth of traveler's checks in Betty's name before leaving for our vacation. This was to make it easy for her to get emergency cash should something serious happen to me on our trip. Now I was confronted with the problem of converting these checks back to cash by having her sign them. And for some unexplainable reason I had purchased most of these in $20 denominations. What a herculean task I had created for her as a result of what I had supposed to be protective planning. I suppose there would have been an easier way, but I accepted this as a challenge of her ability to write her name.

Fortunately the paralysis was only in her left hand, so my problem was limited to getting her to sign her name with her normal writing hand. And I soon learned that words to be written come from the same area of the brain as words to be spoken. After showing her the original signature on the checks, I had her practice copying it several times on a blank piece of paper. It was not long before she could make an acceptable signature, but the letters were made very slowly and painstakingly. Over a period of about a week she was able to sign all the checks, but since she tired quickly from the effort I asked her for only four or five each day. The teller at our local bank, when made aware of her condition, obligingly cashed the checks without witnessing the signature.

Formal speech therapy started at Henry Ford Hospital under the direction of Josephine Simonson only one week after Betty's return from Beaumont Hospital. I had been referred to Miss Simonson by our physician, and when I talked to her on the telephone she agreed to an appointment and felt that she could fit Betty into her schedule. This was indeed fortunate, for there is a scarcity of capable speech therapists trained to meet the need for rehabilitating the many stroke and accident victims afflicted with aphasia. And I have learned that the role of the speech therapist is most important in the process of relearning words. Under the most favorable conditions, and even with a highly motivated patient, the progress would be impossibly slow without the help of a competent therapist.

Ford Hospital is in the inner core of metropolitan Detroit, about eight miles from our suburban home; so getting Betty there and back daily was going to be a problem. At least it seemed that way to me. Driving her own car was out of the question at this stage, and public transportation was not close enough at either end. Taxicabs were a possibility, and so was my housekeeper as a last resort. But I hadn't counted on the great reservoir of human kindness that would start flowing from her friends and neighbors, as well as relatives. Very soon we had enough volunteers to drive her the first week; and then two good friends offered to share the job of scheduling drivers for each coming week. One of them would phone me on Saturday or Sunday and tell me who would do the driving on each day of the next week. I would then make a written schedule to put on our kitchen bulletin board for Betty to use as a reference. There would be a different woman each day, and usually the same person would not drive again for two or three weeks.

I have a list of names of the twenty-five women who participated in this program and their contribution to Betty's progress was inestimable. The fact that her morale was boosted by knowing that so many people were willing to give three hours a day to drive her through city traffic in all kinds of weather was important, although this was not the only benefit. Being with people she knew who would talk to her in spite of her handicap, gave her a feeling of participating, even if only in a small way. I am sure she looked forward each day to meeting one of her friends, and this thread of socializing provided a nourishing tie with the mainstream of life, tending to minimize the feeling of isolation that smothers the initiative of so many aphasics.

A very thorough examination of Betty's hearing capability was made before she was permitted to enter into speech therapy. This surprised me and seemed unnecessary, for I had noticed no deficiency in hearing during our daily confrontation at meal times or during other communication encounters. On the contrary, she seemed overly sensitive to sound. The importance of the hearing examination became clear and meaningful to me only as time went on and I learned that speech therapy for the aphasic involves shadings of sound that have become habitual to the normal person. The hearing examination made use of the most modern equipment and techniques for evaluating the full range capability of both ears, and was conducted by an experienced audiologist. No deterioration of Betty's hearing ability was found.

Likewise she was put through a series of tests to determine the level of her language ability. This provided the speech therapist with specific knowledge of the extent of aphasia in the patient, and formed the basis for projecting the future lesson program.

Miss Simonson lost no time in getting started on the formal speech program and I was most impressed with her understanding of aphasia and her dedication to helping people so afflicted. She immediately established a rapport with Betty that was beautiful to see. I am sure that her inspirational leadership played an important role in Betty's progress. And this is not to detract one bit from the determination and courage on Betty's part that were the other necessary ingredients in this battle of the bottled-up words.

Rarely was I permitted in the room while the lesson was in progress. The few times that I drove Betty to Ford Hospital I waited in the eighth floor lobby until Miss Simonson's door opened an hour later, signaling the end of the session. And I realized that this was right, even though I was consumed with curiosity. The therapist, to be effective, must have the patient's complete attention, and vice versa; and a typical weakness of the aphasic is difficulty concentrating in the pres-

32

ence of even minor distractions. Miss Simonson was well aware of my interest and was very thoughtful in always giving me a complete report of the day's progress as we chatted in her office following the session. She also indicated the things I should do at home with Betty to be of help on the next lesson. She was careful to avoid the reference to what I *could* do at home to help. She put it in a more positive form and referred to things that I *should* do.

She would also write little references in the lesson notebook that was brought home each day, such as "Have Mr. Knox ask you to say the following words to him, and add other words having similar vowel sounds." And so it was that I soon found myself to be a third member of the team.

Homework was assigned each day and Betty worked on her lesson every spare moment—which was practically all of the time when she was not eating or taking her afternoon nap. And with such a display of fortitude and determination, how could I deny her request for help in the evening? It wasn't always the thing I wanted most to do, after one of those hard days at the office, but the hardship was so minor compared to what she was enduring that it wasn't difficult to become reconciled to my role. Furthermore, the sound of television, radio, or hi-fi was unbearable to her at this early stage so I refrained from these forms of entertainment. Betty and I would work together at a table in the den or kitchen while Berniece went upstairs to her room to read, listen to the radio, or watch an old television set that I had moved into her room.

Betty was so persistent in getting help from whatever source was available that she soon had Berniece working with her, usually for a period in the morning and again in the afternoon. Berniece entered into it willingly and was happy to be of help whenever she could. In spite of the shortcomings on the part of both Berniece and myself as speech therapists, we probably were able to help Betty considerably, especially as we learned more about the process of relearning to use language in both speech and writing.

Very few of us remember how we, as individuals, learned to read, write and talk, and I certainly could not be counted among those few. In my association with aphasia it was most difficult for me to learn and master the dual premise that speech is related only to sound (disregarding lip reading), and writing is related to the sight of letters or symbols.

Therefore identifying the word for the patient by means of pantomime or pointing to the physical object has no relationship to an aphasic's process of learning to speak or write. To my chagrin this was impressed upon me many times. One can describe and define an object in all possible ways, but this does not help the patient to speak the word. He usually knows what the object is and you are probably insulting his intelligence when you define it for him, when all he wants to do is pronounce or write the word. This breakdown in communication is extremely frustrating to the patient and, of course, in a lesser degree to a well-meaning but untrained teacher.

Early in the second week of therapy I purchased a tape recorder at the suggestion of Miss Simonson so that she could make use of her department tape recorder to project the daily lesson into our home. Sometimes she would make a tape of her voice directed to

Betty, requesting her to repeat certain sounds and words that were relevant to the current phase of therapy. We would then play the tape on our machine and use the sound of her voice as the subject of a practice session. At other times she would make a tape of the conversation that took place in her office during the lesson that day, and Betty would have an opportunity to hear her own voice responding to that of Miss Simonson. This was most helpful and Betty would become self-critical, using such descriptive words as "lousy" or "messy" to describe her performance. Where these words came from, or how they came through the brain barrier, I have no idea. But it was Miss Simonson's contention from the beginning that the words were all stored away in the brain, and it was our job to develop new channels through which they might be released.

Therapy started with fundamental vowel sounds such as *ow* in *cow* and *how,* and *ou* in *out* and *house.* The sound given by the therapist was always immediately related to writing the word and using it in a sentence. To illustrate: *ow,* as in *cow,* was further presented in the written and spoken sentence, "A cow gives milk." Certainly lip reading, from a clear and exaggerated pronunciation, played a part in learning speech. Even today Betty will ask me to look at her, or she will make a positive effort to watch my lips if she doesn't understand me the first time.

Another marvelous aid to speech improvement is the Language Master. This is an electronic device into which the patient feeds a card. As the card is automatically transferred through the machine, a man's voice from the attached loud speaker booms out the noun that is printed clearly on the card. In addition, the spoken and printed noun is illustrated by a picture on the card. As the patient becomes more proficient, there are more advanced cards that picture an action that is described by a printed sentence. Such a card might have a picture of a boy rolling a hoop, and underneath would be the printed sentence, "The boy is rolling a hoop." The magnetic tape fastened to the card would carry the voice which repeats the sentence in sound. In this type of therapy, lip reading can play no part whatsoever. Further, the electronic aid is so dramatic that most patients find it very exciting, and are eager to participate in this kind of therapy.

In a short time Betty was spending a half hour or more at the Language Master machine, following the one hour session in Miss Simonson's office. She would feed the cards in and, operating it by herself, would become so absorbed that often her driver had to remind her when it was time to leave for home. In the future, we may be certain that dramatic progress will continue in the development and application of scientific aids to speech therapy.

During the period of learning to associate vowel sounds with words and their spelling I recall vividly how certain sounds were readily picked up by Betty and repeated much more easily than others. An example of this is the word *bamboo,* which was one of those words used to illustrate the vowel sound of *oo.* As we would go over a list of words on the lesson page, when the word *bamboo* appeared it would come out like a flash, and clear as a bell—BAM-BOO. I suppose there is a certain drama to this and other sounds related to alliteration that makes them attractive.

Living our lives, at this point, did not go as smoothly

as I have pictured it. There were down periods as well as up periods for both of us. We discontinued attending church, not only because Sunday morning was given over to speech work, but because Betty shrank from exposing her handicap to strange people or even to casual acquaintances. She would not even go for a walk in daylight, so we limited our walking for exercise to hours after dark. Our social life, as we knew it before, disintegrated to the point of nonexistence.

Periodically her morale would plummet to the pit of despair, usually in the late evening when fatigue had set in. Sometimes it occurred when she would suddenly become aware of the void in our social life. During these tearful periods of depression she would say, "Dead, dead," and it was quite clear that she was wishing that the stroke had taken her life. She had been an extremely active person with a long list of community, church, and charitable activities to which she gave a great deal of her time and energy. At the time of the stroke the most important of these was her responsibility as Chairman of the Library Board, a culmination of her life's work as a librarian. So it is not surprising that a sudden withdrawal, for such a busy person, would create a terrible void. The fiercely burning desire to regain her high plateau of participation in community and cultural affairs probably drove her to endure the long hours of work on word therapy.

It was in the early part of this initial period of therapy that she reached for the Bible one night as we lay in bed waiting and hoping to be drugged into sleep by our pills. Betty had found it necessary to use one pill for sleep long before the stroke, and even now she carefully limited herself to only one upon retiring. I had been one of those fortunate people who are dead to the world almost immediately after hitting the bed, but now I too required help from the pill bottle.

When she handed me the Bible and said, "pray," I knew she meant for me to read the Lord's Prayer, so she could follow the words as I read them. As I repeated the familiar words she occasionally would say after me a word that was recalled. Thus began the lesson that continued nightly until, many months later, Betty was able to repeat the Lord's Prayer reasonably well from memory with a minimum of prompting. I would hold the passage from the sixth chapter of Matthew in front of us and read slowly, while she followed by reading and listening at first, and later she would say the words with me. But there was a deeper meaning to this than just learning the words of the Lord's Prayer. She felt the need for help and spiritual strength that she could get only from the Almighty. And I too found that prayer, either silent or spoken, was a source of strength that sustained me in my moments of discouragement.

As the spring season advanced and nature slowly burst its bonds of winter, the effort that Betty was putting into her work started to produce some small rewards and my hopes for a recovery grew almost daily. One Sunday in the middle of May we drove to Ann Arbor for a dual birthday celebration with two of our grandchildren. The selecting of birthday gifts which was normally done by Betty now required help and direction from me, but she had participated as best she could.

As we drove along I decided to find out if she could sing the words to the "Happy Birthday" tune. Such a demonstration would be a surprise for our son and would give Grandma a more normal posture for the children. She responded to the suggestion enthusiastically, hummed the tune immediately, and in a very short time was singing the words. It was a happy day for both of us and I could sense that her morale was boosted by the feeling of accomplishment.

It is probably difficult to appreciate how such a simple achievement could be considered an important milestone of early progress. It amounted to the repeating of only four words and the names of two grandchildren, but compared to her level of accomplishment in speech therapy, consisting of repeating of simple isolated words, this was indeed a rewarding experience. Miss Simonson had commented that words associated with a musical rhythm were most readily recalled by aphasics. So the "Happy Birthday" episode was followed soon by other limited successes with "Onward Christian Soldiers" and other tunes similarly rooted in the distant past.

3

Lightning Strikes Again

Friday, May 22, was a day of personal accomplishment for me. Certain important engineering projects in which I had played a significant role were appoaching fruition. I had completed dictating a summary report and felt that it would be well received. So it was with a light heart that I made my customary weekly stop at our local bank on my trip home that night. I had reflected on Betty's progress and I looked forward to our review of her lesson and her trip to Ford Hospital with her friend, Lou Van Camp. Even the weather made its contribution to this feeling of well-being. A gentle warm breeze had teamed with a bright sun and cloudless sky to produce a perfect spring day.

I drove into the side drive confidently, with not the slightest hint of any impending disaster. Before I could open the car door Berniece burst from the house and quietly but excitedly informed me that something was wrong with Betty. She was not communicating in any way and had been this way since her afternoon nap. Berniece wanted to catch me before I went into the house so I would be prepared for the change. I wouldn't let myself believe it was as serious as Berniece implied, but when I confronted Betty seated on the sofa and received no response—nothing but a silent stare—I knew the worst had happened. The animation of her greeting —which I had come to expect in recent weeks—was gone. I talked to her but there was no response except an occasional negative shake of the head. I tried to interest her in the words of the current lesson written in her notebook. No response. I asked her what had happened. A shrug of the shoulders. She was able to walk and there seemed to be no paralysis, but I knew she had experienced a repetition of the initial damaging episode.

Berniece related that when Betty and Mrs. Van Camp had returned from the hospital earlier in the afternoon they were both bubbling with enthusiasm and Mrs. Van Camp joked and spoke animatedly. Her titillating vitality seemed to transfer to Betty contagiously. Shortly after, Betty had gone upstairs for her regular afternoon nap (or rest). About an hour later Berniece heard her get up and go into the bathroom. Some time later she had come downstairs in the confused state that I now found her.

I described Betty's condition and the related events to the doctor over the telephone, but he apparently did not consider her in need of emergency treatment and did not come to examine her until the following afternoon. After his examination, which involved conversation with her and the testing of certain reflexes, he said everything seemed to indicate that she had experienced another stroke. He made an appointment for her to see the neurologist at Beaumont Hospital the following Monday.

That weekend is indelibly imprinted in my memory. I had never experienced defeat as crushing as this. When I thought of the hours of courageous effort that she had put into the struggle against her conversation-crippling handicap, only to have it nullified in a few seconds, I was overwhelmed with despair. And if I felt this way, what could be going through her mind? She was certainly suffering the impact of this blow more than I was, yet there was no outward sign of mental depression at this point. Only silence and a complete lack of communication.

My older brother came to see us Saturday afternoon, and as he and I left the living room where he had been talking to Betty and trying to cheer her up, I was completely overcome by my pent-up emotions and started to sob uncontrollably. He immediately admonished me not to let Betty see me that way, and I knew he was right. After giving relief to my feelings behind the closed kitchen door I pulled myself together and poured each of us a bracing drink. That seemed to be a turning point. I knew I must continue to show Betty that my confidence in her recovery was as strong as ever. I had told her before, and would continue to tell her, that together we would win this fight. Now, more than ever, she would need the strength that would flow from my outward show of confidence. I remembered incidents from my earlier life related to lesser illnesses, and how I had been buoyed by the presence of a cheerful person. The negative or neutral personality is remembered as a great big nothing. The cheerful person with the smiling and confident aspect had been a source of strength and courage. Certainly all professional medical practitioners know this age-old truth and use it as a professional tool. So why wouldn't my use of this proven patient psychology be a most effective way of helping Betty? I would be with her every day, whereas a doctor is more limited in his time with a patient.

For those people who are normally outgoing and cheerful, it is quite natural to present this air of optimism most of the time. It is my nature to be more withdrawn and introspective—to look upon life too seriously. So it has taken real effort to attempt this change in my personality. I have not always succeeded, but the effort seems worthwhile.

I accompanied Betty to Beaumont Hospital the following Monday where she was examined by the staff specialist in neurology. Thursday of that week, under his direction, she was given an electroencephalogram (EEG) test, which produces a printed tape of electrical impulses from various sections of the brain. No special preparation of the patient is required for this, so she completed it as an outpatient in the laboratory.

Saturday of that week was Memorial Day and I recall listening to the Indianapolis 500-mile race on the radio outdoors because the noise and crowd excitement bothered Betty. I was glad to have this as a distraction from my inner thoughts, and to familiarize myself with current sports events so I could participate in conversation with my business associates at lunch the following Monday. More and more I was conscious of becoming an outsider to the group, unable to contribute to the daily discussion of current happenings.

Apparently the EEG test did not provide a complete description of what had happened, for on the following Tuesday, June 2, I accompanied Betty to another test.

This was much more sophisticated than previous tests but required, as preparation, only the injection of medication a few hours in advance. The medication was a chemical compound containing a radioactive isotope, and was selected for its characteristic of seeking out and collecting at the sites of brain damage. When it has come to rest in the area where damage has occurred it continues to send out radiation energy in all directions. By suitable detection means it is possible to make a map of the damaged area. The patient is carefully and precisely located in a prone position such that the sensing device can be traversed slowly back and forth, hori-- zontally, in a straight line above the patient's head. The motion of the sensing device is not continuous but rather a series of short start-and-stop movements. During this traverse the radiation impulses impinge on a sensitized paper which has been treated in such a way that a black dot appears where the beam of radiation strikes. Where there is no radiated beam of energy, no dot appears. A series of parallel lines, closely spaced, is traversed to provide a broad picture of the damaged area. Any region of the map that is blackened by the dots is a damaged region.

A repetition of this procedure with the patient's head in several positions is necessary to produce a three-dimensional diagram of the affected area of the brain. Since this entire program is fundamentally similar to a photographic technique, the patient is required to refrain from moving for a considerable period of time.

I sat alongside the apparatus and watched the entire procedure, marveling all the while at what man had wrought in this beneficial application of nuclear science. It was a stirring demonstration of three disciplines—science, engineering, and medicine—combining to produce a useful tool of civilization.

The results of this test, commonly called a brain scan, confirmed that the speech area of the brain had again been damaged by a vascular accident; but following a consultation a short time later between the neurologist, the neurosurgeon, and our doctor, it was decided to hospitalize Betty to repeat the arteriogram and the pneumoencephalogram procedures that were done in March. I was at a loss to understand why this was necessary, since I had seen the charts resulting from the brain scan which seemed to confirm brain damage in the speech area. But it was explained that they still had not determined the precise cause of the brain damage. This decision was hard for me to take, for I knew how difficult it would be for Betty to go back into the hospital and to endure the suffering of those two test procedures again. However, she took the decision in stride and was apparently willing to do almost anything that offered some hope for improving her condition.

About this time some of my friends spoke knowledgeably of acquaintances who had suffered a single stroke and then experienced a second and sometimes a third stroke. The repeat strokes had not been as severe as the first and they presumed that such an eventuality was not uncommon and should not be unexpected. I suppose they thought that somehow this would make me feel better about what had happened—that Betty wasn't so different after all.

Betty was hospitalized on June 9 and it was at this time that our doctor hinted to me that something more serious than the common stroke might have occurred.

He spoke of Pick's disease and described it in dire terms, explaining that it causes a gradual shrinking of the brain over a long period, which results in progressive brain damage and mental deterioration. Inasmuch as there is no known cure, he hoped they would find no confirmation of this in the arteriogram or the pneumo-encephalogram. I was horrified at this monstrous possibility.

The week of suspense waiting for the completion of these tests seemed unending, and made the period of waiting for the birth of a first child seem riotously happy and short by comparison. I worked at my job, but little was accomplished. I called the doctor the day following the final diagnostic procedure and he suggested that I call him the next afternoon following a scheduled meeting with the neurosurgeon. I called him promptly from my office and, following the usual delay in reaching a doctor, he came to the telephone and delivered the blow. He said it was the opinion of the neurosurgeon that Betty had Pick's disease.

Although the doctor continued to talk I was too stunned to hear. Finally I managed, "Can you explain how the neurosurgeon reached such a conclusion?" He said there were several factors that tied together, but the keystone in the arch of evidence was the revelation that the space between the skull and the outer surface of the brain appeared to have grown slightly larger during the short span of time between March and June— indicating a probable shrinkage of the brain.

I know practically nothing of the surgical procedures on which this opinion was based, so I felt privileged, as well as obliged, to question whether their degree of accuracy warranted a positive conclusion. I asked for a meeting with the neurosurgeon and it was arranged. In no mood to continue working at my job that day, I went home sorrowful and disheartened.

The following day Janet and David Jr. joined me at the hospital for the meeting with the neurosurgeon. He was properly sympathetic and understanding of our desire to have another medical opinion, and said he would submit all of the hospital charts and records to whomever we selected. We discussed some neurosurgeons in the Detroit area, but David was strongly in favor of taking his mother to University Hospital in Ann Arbor where both the supporting staff and the available diagnostic techniques were superb.

With very little further discussion we agreed to arrange an appointment with the top neurosurgeon at University Hospital. Understandably, we had not told Betty of the Beaumont diagnosis. She was told that it had not yet been satisfactorily determined what caused the second loss of speech, and it was our recommendation that she should go to University Hospital where there were more experienced doctors and the most advanced diagnostic aids. We were careful to have her approval and understanding.

Our first trip to Ann Arbor was fruitless, since the doctor had been called out of town on an emergency only an hour before our arrival. However, one of his staff assistants gave Betty a brief examination. Our second visit about a week later also came to nothing because the Beaumont records had not been received. Finally on July 7 Betty was given a thorough examination by the neurosurgeon. He decided that another brain scan should be made immediately.

After observing the brain scan procedure in the labo-

48

ratory once more, I took Betty to the lobby for the long wait for a call from the doctor. It was late afternoon when it came. After directing us into his private office he dramatically pointed to two charts temporarily hung on the wall with adhesive tape.

He said, "That one with the darkened damaged area of the brain was made at Beaumont Hospital in early June, one month ago. Now look at the other one that was made here today. That same area now is entirely clear. No further damage has occurred since she had the second stroke. She should start speech therapy again as quickly as possible."

"Do you mean?" I started, but did not finish as he interrupted with, "That's exactly what I mean. She's going to be fine and you should get her into the speech therapy program immediately."

I was floating on air after hearing these words and thanked him profusely as we left. Since it is now more than five years since that prophetic statement, and nothing but progressive improvement has occurred since, I have the highest regard for that doctor's skill and judgment.

After telephoning the good news to our children in Ann Arbor I drove home in a happy frame of mind. As difficult as the days ahead would certainly be, now there was hope in the place of despair.

4

Living Adjustments

Although I was buoyed by the new turn of events and anticipated the beginning of speech therapy again, the specter of "that other disease" lurked in the remote recesses of my mind for many months. This gnawing doubt probably contributed to my growing condition of poor health—increased nervousness and loss of weight.

I had kept Miss Simonson informed of what was going on at Beaumont Hospital and University Hospital and she was delighted to welcome Betty back into speech therapy the Monday following the Ann Arbor diagnosis. The speech lessons started again with the basic phonetic sounds, only this time the rate of learning was slower than before. In a telephone conversation I had with Miss Simonson she said the aphasia was much deeper in the speech regions this time, and it would take a great deal of effort and time for Betty to get back to where she was in May. As was done before, she was given a complete series of tests to determine her abilities before starting the program of speech rehabilitation.

Once again the local ladies provided transportation to Ford Hospital for Betty, only this time the Huntington Woods Study Club, a women's cultural group of which Betty had once served as president, made a project of the job of transporting her, and assigned a responsible chairman. What a wonderful help this arrangement was! The ladies carried it off like clockwork, through good weather and bad, and provided timely replacements when illness interfered. Not once was Betty late for a lesson, nor did she miss an appointment for lack of transportation.

We soon settled down to the routine of home assignments again, but now the homework was more extensive. Miss Simonson found it necessary to limit the lessons to three days a week, so the home assignments covered two nights instead of just one. I worked with her each night and as much as possible on weekends. She would become exhausted, and it was evident that a great deal of energy was used up in the mental process of relearning to speak and understand words and sentences.

Some nights I was painfully aware that she was making no progress, that she seemed to be standing still. What I thought she had accomplished the night before was lost, and we would go over it again and again. I would become discouraged and try as I would to keep from showing it, I am sure she sensed my depression. This would last perhaps a few days and suddenly she would leap forward in a burst of progress and the world would seem right again. Miss Simonson would confirm this upward acceleration to me in one of our periodic telephone conversations, saying that Betty was really running with the words again. She said she had noticed this phenomenon of step progress in other patients, and we should expect it as a normal situation.

Almost immediately after starting speech therapy again we began to go out to restaurants for Sunday dinner. With Betty's help I would prepare the dinner Saturday night after Berniece had left for the weekend, but I rebelled on Sunday. The problem with eating out was the exposure to people, and the irritation resulting from the noise. But on Sunday I was able to find a few restaurants that were quiet enough to satisfy her. However, she would select a table in a corner, if available, as far as possible from other people and preferably adjacent to empty tables. If I remained quiet and provided no conversation she would become self-conscious and urge me to say something ("Talk, talk!") so that people nearby would not suspect there was something wrong with her. This extreme sensitivity to people-exposure gradually lessened as time went on; but even today, after five years, Betty prefers to dine in a quiet atmosphere.

One of our early visits to a restaurant was to celebrate a birthday, and the party included her two sisters and their husbands. Unfortunately I had neglected to specify a table location when I made the reservation. We were directed to a table directly in front of the piano just as the musical combo swung into the noisiest section of their performance. Betty put her hands to her ears and backed away, saying, "I can't, I can't." We finally obtained a table at the opposite end of the room. We have returned to this restaurant many times since, but we always find a table some distance from the music.

Sensitivity to surroundings is not limited to the noise level. Betty has always been a neat person and has kept our home clean and orderly, even during the trying period when the children were small. In those days, however, she tempered her need for order and cleanliness for the sake of overall effectiveness as a mother and housewife. After her stroke, however, the slightest blemish became an intense irritant. Windows had to be washed more frequently. If my necktie was slightly askew, if a tiny piece of lint showed on my coat, she would call my attention to these or any other imperfections and have me correct them before leaving the house. A drop of water on the kitchen floor, a tiny spot of soil on the carpet, a picture on the wall sightly askew —all were glaring eyesores and had to be eliminated.

Nor was this sensitivity to surroundings limited to indoors. A small piece of windblown paper on the lawn or leaves littering the sidewalk received her immediate attention. Providentially, her shortness of memory often permitted us to postpone immediate action. Out of sight was out of mind, but the irritation would be repeated often enough to require eventual corrective action.

It seemed to me that this greater sensitivity to what I like to call the "little things" might be a counteraction to her affliction as a result of frustration, a subconscious insistence on perfection in other things to offset the imperfection in her speech. Miss Simonson told me she had noticed this increased sensitivity in most of her aphasic patients and considered it a common characteristic of people so afflicted. She was interested to hear me confirm this and felt that I should not be overly concerned. So I soon learned to adjust to this slight aberration of personality.

It was November 8, 1964, when Betty finally agreed to attend a Sunday church service. The selection of attire proved to be a real problem and was one of the early evidences of difficulty in decision making which is probably generally characteristic of aphasics. She was very conscious of her appearance and was painfully anxious to look her best before others. She had tried on two outfits and then went back to the first again when I entered the room and exclaimed how attractive she looked in that one. Apparently that remark made her decision easier, but such complimentary statements by me did not always produce a firm decision.

Upon arriving at the church she insisted that we sit near the rear of the sanctuary and in seats that were closest to the side aisle. If the usher showed others to our pew, she would cling to the aisle seats and let the others squeeze by us to reach the middle seats. This preference, I believe, was related to a fear of a new or unexpected situation, a fear of something happening to her requiring a quick exit—a kind of claustrophobia. Being near the rear of the congregation also had to do with minimum exposure to people both during the service and as we left the church.

Fear and nervousness showed in her face that first time and I would occasionally nudge her reassuringly. I took great pride in her church attendance as evidence of her progress and her indomitable spirit. Occasionally tears would well up in my eyes during the singing of a hymn as the emotional impact of her struggle to become normal broke down my unruffled calm exterior. I am sure that some of the early sermons were beyond her grasp, but she seemed to get comfort from the quiet period of prayer and the singing of the hymns. I would shudder for her when the prelude of organ music would suddenly become loud and overpowering. The proper rendition of the Bach prelude on that first Sunday morning apparently required such a crescendo, but Betty withstood the sound onslaught with no apparent ill effects. As time went on she became more tolerant of the exposure to people. It was not long before she would want to sit on the center aisle occasionally so we could join the line of people to greet the minister as we went out of the sanctuary.

As the lessons proceeded following Betty's second stroke, Miss Simonson called my attention to one of the marks of progress we should look for. In the early stages of speech therapy Betty would try to repeat the word spoken to her and would look for a sign of approval or disapproval as a measure of her success. But after about six or eight weeks she started to show an increased awareness of the sound her voice was making and to make a comparison between this sound and the sound and inflection of the teacher's voice. This is called monitoring by the professional, and was what we had been eagerly anticipating. After Betty fully reached the stage of monitoring, her progress was much more rapid. She now could repeat some of the lesson words by herself, and know if they were spoken correctly. More often than not, however, she would know that she had said the word incorrectly, and needed a helper to put her back on the track.

During the first six months the tantrums that would seize her on rare occasions were a reminder of the severity of the frustrations filling her life. Often the frustration was over a little word. Before she had firmly fixed the distinction between the words "yes" and "no," she would sometimes say "yes" when she meant "no," and vice versa. One day my misunderstanding of her intent with respect to which restaurant she preferred arose from the misuse of "yes" and "no," and triggered a tantrum directed against me. Such an occurrence was an extreme departure from our former relationship and I was understandably shaken. I had to learn, over a period of time, to cope with this by being patient and substituting love for angry reaction. This did not come easily, for it involved the realization that she was not quite the same person during these periods, and gradually I had to bring her back to her normal posture. It also involved the realization that my personality trait of reacting too quickly needed some overhauling. Following the recovery of her composure—and mine—I would tell her what I was to repeat many times, that she was going to win this fight, that together we could overcome her loss of speech, and she would once more talk with people.

It was in this early period that I became extremely apprehensive, and I suppose it was related to the stress associated with her illness and the impact of a harsh new way of life for me. I became overly sensitive to any little unusual noise which I imagined as a potential threat, and the sudden unexpected blare of a car horn while driving startled me with fear of an impending accident.

While shaving in the morning I would listen subconsciously for any indication of disturbance in our routine. With the radio on, while listening to the morning news, I would imagine I heard her calling "Dave! Dave!" With heart pounding I would turn off the radio, half expecting some indication of fire, a fall downstairs or some similar catastrophe. The ensuing silence was always reassuring.

While walking with her outside one evening I smelled smoke and immediately concluded it was coming from our house. I ran home as quickly as possible and was greatly relieved to find that all was well. I was also chagrined, for had I been my normal self I would have known that a neighbor's incinerator was burning trash and would not have given it a second thought.

I lost weight in this period and did not sleep well. I had gotten into the habit of having two drinks as I read the evening paper before dinner. This gave me a pleasant interlude between my workday at the office and my workday at home, and seemed to provide the proper preparation for eating. But I found myself drifting into having a brandy or whiskey and then two, as we worked together in the evening on the word lesson. I stopped this as I suddenly realized that I was using it as a crutch, and had probably developed a psychological background that was fertile soil for alcoholism.

Time proved to be the best cure for my nervousness and apprehension. Gradually I adjusted to our new life and by January I was gaining weight, and with a little effort and determination I was able to part with my nightly sleeping pill.

When it came time for the preparation of our Christmas cards that first year she consented, reluctantly, to having most of the envelopes addressed from her list by my business secretary. A few of her close friends were purposely omitted from the list, however, and she insisted on addressing those and even including the usual personal note on many of them. It was necessary for me to compose the notes, but I worked closely with her and tried to treat the task as a supplement to her lessons. Needless to say, we made the most of each personal note that was composed, using many of the same sentences over and over.

In the process of addressing the envelopes many mistakes were made, and she would not permit the envelope to be marred by adding an obvious correction, or by the use of an eraser. So the waste basket started to pile up with discarded envelopes. We found it almost impossible to buy replacement envelopes of the identical size, color, and texture in the local stores. So it was necessary to go back to the source that produced the card to get suitable replacements.

Since that first Christmas she has progressively taken on more of the Christmas card chore herself and now addresses all of them in her own handwriting with a minimum of spoilage. It is still necessary that I help her with the wording of the notes, but from the very first holiday season she has painstakingly made a list of names of those who sent us greeting cards, and preserves this list for reference the following year.

5

Driver's License Renewal

Permitting Betty to drive her car loomed as a hazard to be avoided as long as possible. I was assuming the same attitude toward her driving that I had with our teen-age children—probably for the same reasons. I was not sure if she was capable, at all times, of the judgment that we associate with maturity; and, more importantly, I selfishly shied away from adding another worry to an existence already top-heavy with concern. I knew that her muscular coordination was good. But would she recognize a stop sign, or a no-left-turn sign; and what about recognition of the red and green lights and their implied meaning? What was the possibility of her becoming lost and confused? What would she do if the car stalled, or if a tire went flat, or some other malfunction occurred?

One Sunday afternoon in November, at her insistence, I finally agreed to ride with her in the small car we had bought expressly for her use a year earlier. I asked her to stay within our immediate community and to stay off the bordering traffic arteries. Not knowing what to expect I nervously took the passenger seat on the right as she climbed in behind the wheel. This time I did not forget my safety belt, after making sure that she was buckled up. For the first few blocks I literally hung on, watching her every move and frequently giving her unwanted advice. Then my confidence increased as she negotiated turns handily and stopped at the familiar stop streets. This initial demonstration was soon followed by longer rides and eventually forays onto streets carrying heavier traffic, where she demonstrated that she could react quickly to situations requiring a sudden stop.

It was not long before I was convinced that she was just as skillful and careful a driver as she had always been. When we would approach traffic control lights she would repeat, "Red, stop! Green, go!", but not to identify the significance of the lights. She well knew the significance. She was only practicing the words. But there still remained two hurdles to be cleared before she could drive alone. The first was the renewal of her driver's license which had expired January 10, 1965. The second was to provide a satisfactory way for her to cope with emergency situations.

Anticipating that the local police would want a statement from her doctor, my first step was to get such a statement. The doctor helpfully wrote that there was no medical reason why she should be denied a driver's license. To get her to face up to taking the test was more difficult. After a considerable inner struggle she finally agreed to take the test on a Saturday morning when I could accompany her and provide some moral muscle. One requirement is to pass a vision test. Miss Simonson and I spent considerable time with her on the alphabet, to be more certain that what she spoke would coincide with what she saw. As we walked into the police station she said, softly, "Nervous, nervous!" Of course she was nervous. Aren't we all when we take a driver's license test? What was startling about this exclamation was her ability to make it.

She did quite well with the test. She did well enough to warrant the examining officer to say that she could have her license if she would give a satisfactory driving demonstration on Monday. Her sister, Marion, drove her to the station on Monday, and that evening she greeted me with the temporary driving permit, to be used until the final permit could be issued from Lansing. So now I was faced with the actuality of her driving alone.

I preferred to have her wait until April when the streets would be free of snow and ice, before she drove alone to Henry Ford Hospital for speech therapy. She continued to ride with her regular drivers until some time in March when a few of the ladies agreed to accompany her as a passenger in her car. Understandably there were some who were too timid to trust her driving ability and shied away from such an arrangement. This transition period with the protection of a passenger provided confidence that she could thread her way through city traffic to the hospital without losing her bearings.

Finally the big day came early in April when she was to make the trip alone. This time it was I who was "nervous, nervous." I had provided her with an identification paper on which was typed all the information necessary to help her through any of the emergency situations that might occur.

Identification

My name is Betty Knox.

My speech has been affected by a stroke.

I am taking speech therapy at Henry Ford Hospital.

My home address is 10474 Lincoln, Huntington Woods, Michigan.

My home telephone is 543–0124.

My husband, David Knox, can be reached at Bundy Tubing Co.

His telephone is 536–2580.

My 1962 Chevrolet has complete insurance coverage.

Insurance includes Road Aid. Telephone WO 5–4400.

Insurance identification cards, driver's license, and registration certificate are in my purse.

I am in need of help and would appreciate your assistance in one of the following:

    (1) My car will not start.

    (2) I have a flat tire.

    (3) Please call a taxi for me, and ask him to drive me to:

        (a) Home (address above).

    or

        (b) Henry Ford Hospital. Eighth floor, Miss Simonson, speech therapist.

    (4) Please telephone my home for assistance.

    (5) Please telephone my husband for assistance.

The preparation of this had taken some planning and I felt that it was about as much protection as I could give her, as a driving aphasic. She was to carry it in her purse always and I hoped that it would give me some peace of mind. I had several copies available for her as replacements.

She was due to arrive in Miss Simonson's office at ten o'clock and I called from my office at five minutes after ten. Miss Simonson said she was sitting across the table from her, bright-eyed, safe and sound, and feeling very satisfied with herself. Another milestone!

An interesting corollary to this occurred a few weeks later. Betty had driven to the dry cleaner's with some clothes and when she came out her car would not start. She consulted her identification paper and decided to walk the two blocks to the nearest gas station. While walking she repeated over and over the words from the instruction sheet, "My car will not start," so she would not have to be embarrassed by pointing to the written sentence. The attendant understood her and drove her back to the cleaner's where her car was standing. She then sat in the car and steered as he pushed her to the gas station. Next she telephoned my office to ask me to pick her up, making use of the instruction sheet for the phone number. But it was after 5 P.M., and the answering plant guard told her I had left for home. She then called Berniece at home and somehow made it clear where she was located. Berniece picked her up in her car and drove her home. When I arrived home I was unaware of the ordeal to which Betty had been subjected, and which she had met so courageously and successfully solved; and I was amazed as the entire incident was related to me.

It was encouraging that she had made practical use of my instruction sheet in relating her problem to the gas station attendant, and in making the telephone calls. After that display of dogged determination and ingenuity in taking care of herself, I had no more fear for her in such situations.

6

Speech Laboratory

Long before the anniversary of her stroke in Mexico Betty would say, "One year, talking?" She was voicing a hope, perhaps more than a prediction, that one year of speech therapy would be enough to recover her lost art of conversation. She remembered, as I did, early references of both the doctor and Miss Simonson to "one year at least, and maybe longer" as the necessary time span for speech therapy. Nothing was said that would define the level of accomplishment at the end of that period. It did not occur to me to press for a definition since I could not, or would not, conceive of any level of speech that was in the gray area short of full recovery.

At this point it did not seem possible that Betty would be anywhere near a normal speaking level twelve months after the first stroke. On the other hand I had no way of knowing if there would be a sudden surge of accomplishment after reaching a predictable springboard. Nor did I know if there would be a limit to her potential achievement, in which case the time to reach such a subnormal plateau was also an unknown.

The first time she put the question to me I reminded her that we could not count the word study prior to her second stroke because all of the progress made in that period had been wiped out. We should rightfully consider August 1 as representing the end of one year of speech therapy. She understood the logic of this and seemed satisfied, but the question was repeated more than once because her memory span for recent events was so short.

This seems to be a contradiction. How do we explain her ability to remember the statements about one year of therapy made by the doctor and the speech therapist? She recalled these statements and they were made shortly after her first stroke. I have noticed this memory-selectivity phenomenon many times, and it seems to be related to the importance she attaches to the event. Perhaps there is a limit to the rate of absorbing events into the memory system that is lower for aphasics than for the nonafflicted person. In such case there would be a subconscious tendency to absorb preferentially the more important events and to reject automatically those of lesser importance.

Miss Simonson was noncommittal about the time to reach an acceptable speech level and she was just as noncommittal about the possible limit to the upper level of achievement. She explained that each case of aphasia is an unique situation, and that the end result for Betty was unpredictable at that time. "We should keep working on the program as hard as possible," she indicated, "and as long as we continue to see improvement we will have hope for a high level of recovery."

In the winter of 1965 a few of our good friends, who were also business associates of many years, started to revive for us a pleasant pattern of periodic dinner parties. The thoughtful hostess who first invited us was very kind and understanding, asking first if Betty felt up to having dinner with them and with another couple who were also good friends. She thought it would be good for Betty to get out and have a change of surroundings on a Saturday night, and they would understand if she tired early and wanted to leave. Betty was not yet using the telephone, so I accepted with pleasure, feeling that she was ready for socializing with such a congenial group of old friends. She had some misgivings, but was willing to try it in view of our longstanding friendship with the group.

That dinner proved to be a pivotal point in her progress up the social ladder. Her tolerance of multiple conversations, always a problem for aphasics, was quite good and she made a yeoman's try at making herself understood as best she could with isolated words. I stood close by with one ear cocked toward her conversation and filled in some verbs for her occasionally to keep the conversation moving. All complimented her on how well she was doing which of course gave her a lift even though she politely asked "Sure, sure?"

While cocktails were being served she sipped on a soft drink which she persisted in calling 7-Up, no matter whether it was Coca-cola, ginger-ale, or 7-Up, and this became a by-word for her drinking habits. She was adamant about refraining from taking alcohol, although she had been a mild social drinker before her stroke. I agreed with her wholeheartedly and did not press her to take a drink. I am not sure if this was entirely her decision or if Miss Simonson had talked to her. Certainly it was a sound decision, for the aphasic has difficulty enough with words while completely sober, without compounding the situation with alcohol.

Each subsequent dinner party brought forth comments on how well she was progressing with her conversational speech. The span of time between dinners was great enough to register a noticeable change for our friends, whereas, my daily observation did not permit ready recognition of the steady sweep of progress. These get-togethers enabled me to put her level of achievement in perspective, though vicariously, and they gave both of us the opportunity to get away from our tedious treadmill for a pleasant interlude.

Although we were not able to reciprocate by entertaining at home, both of us were eager to continue socializing with our friends and felt that we should carry our share of the entertainment responsibility. So when our turn came we took the group to a reasonably quiet restaurant for dinner, after first entertaining them with cocktails in our home.

These dinners were quite widely spaced in time, but other social opportunities gradually started to present themselves as word got around that Betty was able to enjoy the company of our friends again. A group of her sorority sisters and their husbands with whom we had enjoyed semiannual, potluck dinners for a number of years, invited us to join them again. She felt quite comfortable in the company of these girlfriends of long standing, in spite of her shortcomings in speech. Someday soon we hope she will feel up to hostessing this group once more, although it has not yet been possible.

Two widow ladies whose husbands had been friends of mine, and who had come to know Betty very well, graciously provided a dinner outing on two occasions, and each time Betty showed more poise and tolerance for strange surroundings. Another occasion for social exposure was a wedding on May 8, 1965, in which our daughter Margaret was maid of honor. This was quite a test for Betty because, although the bride was a close friend of our daughter, we were acquainted with very few of the guests. She knew very well the social amenities of a wedding, but it took a lot of courage to go through the reception line.

I came to realize more and more the value of increasing exposure to people in a conversational framework. In the cloistered and casual atmosphere of the therapist's workroom the patient may rise to heights that are very encouraging to the therapist and quite satisfying to the patient. But it remains a question whether the patient will make an equally good showing with the newly acquired speech skill under the social pressures of a group. Certainly a degree of success in the group, and a recognizable acceptance by the group, generates self-confidence in the patient, and this self-confidence may be important to the aphasic's progress. The feeling of inferiority and the tendency to withdraw appear to be strong forces and may be overcome by the strength which grows from confidence. And confidence can be generated from practice and repeated success.

Just as the spring season signals the cyclical renewal of all nature, so it creates in the hearts of women a yearning for a new look for the nest—even after the young have long since taken flight. The sofa in the living room was, as she put it, "messy" and "lousy" that spring, and I had to agree she was right. So here was an opportunity for her to practice judgment, decision making, and meaningful conversation related to a major household purchase. She had already experienced the exposure to sales people in buying a dress for herself and, aside from some procrastination in deciding which garment she preferred, there were no problems. We found that, generally, the older sales clerks are very understanding of the speech handicap. Once they are aware of the condition they will listen patiently and, when necessary, look to the husband for clarification.

I learned very early that, although Betty needed and wanted me with her when making a purchase, she was insistent on carrying on the conversation with the clerk by herself, and called on me for help only when she was in deep trouble. This was another demonstration of the importance of learning by doing, and thereby gaining confidence as well as competence.

After we had looked at sofas in a preliminary survey of the local stores, a friend suggested that a neighbor, whom I shall call Jean, might help us. We had known Jean and her husband before his death, but were not aware that she was now a specialist in a furniture store. Having a sales person who was a former acquaintance was helpful to Betty at this stage. On each visit to the store she would ask for Jean, as she felt comfortable with her. It took but two visits to decide on the style and make of sofa, but the selection of the upholstering was something else.

Jean finally furnished her with a group of sample fabrics to take home and study for a week, and to compare with the other colors in our room. I was of no help to her and she well knew that my color judgment could not be trusted. I inherited that color confusion, so common among males, that is called color blindness.

Any one of several of the swatches would have been

an excellent selection, and she quickly narrowed the choice to two or three. Now she had entered the decision-making stage, which proved to be most difficult. She seemed to be extremely sensitive to the possibility of making an error of judgment, and vacillated from one choice to another. She got Berniece's preference. She got her older sister's preference. She got her younger sister's preference.

Since there was considerable concurrence between these preferences and her apparent liking, she at last made a decision. Her selection was superb, it had both a pleasing harmony with the carpet coloring and a long-wearing characteristic.

An aphasic is uncertain of himself and his judgment. He has been severely shaken by what has happened to him. He needs help and encouragement, and looks hungrily for commendation to strengthen his confidence. We should give it to him as often as possible, and then we should repeat it, for his memory is short.

Illustrating how normally feminine her thinking was, Betty couldn't possibly visualize a crisp new sofa in the same room with those "messy" looking drapes. And she was able to convey her opinion to me in no uncertain terms. Further, that upholstered chair near the front window was "sad." I assured her that I did not disagree, and that we would start immediately to look at materials for new drapes, and then we would pick out a new fabric for recovering the chair. The sofa was more than two months in coming, but this period was occupied with drape and chair therapy, and of course we had a painter cover the living room walls with a fresh coat of paint, a lighter shade than the old color in keeping with the interior decorating trend of that period.

She entered into the redecorating project with so much enthusiasm that it was readily apparent that she needed this kind of diversional activity to take her mind from her formal speech work. This was recreation for her, but it was also a kind of creative work which permitted her to have a sense of achievement in a field of endeavor apart from speech. Yet the entire redecorating project was interwoven with opportunities for vocal self-expression. Even after completion, each redecorated object became a focal point for conversation.

Although activity related to such a project as interior decorating is generated by the patient, she needs help in completing the details. It took a great deal of my spare time to accompany her on shopping expeditions devoted to redecorating the living room. I also spent shopping time with her in the selection of her personal attire. If I had followed my normal inclination and played golf, or read books, or pursued my other hobbies, I would have been a very unhappy man, knowing that I had denied Betty one of the avenues to self-expression and recovery. Working together was an unspoken expression of love which carried with it multiple compensations. For her these compensations were mental exhilaration, recreation, and self-expression; for me they were gratification with her progress, and an overwhelming sense of purpose in life.

She revived another recreational activity by starting to knit again, commencing with a rather simple knit dishcloth. She made many of these for her friends and for the church bazaar. Although Betty had previously been an accomplished knitter and had produced many sweaters of complicated design for the American Field Service and for her own use, her stroke had wiped out this talent as well as the ability to read and follow complicated instructions. So she was limited to the simple forms at first, but fortunately she had no serious paralysis that would prevent this manual activity. I believe the slight paralysis that she did have in her left hand was benefited by her knitting as a form of physical therapy.

When she tired of the monotony of square dishcloths, she resurrected an old set of instructions for making a child's knitted ball, and proceeded to make a large number of these toy balls for grandchildren and friends. Although her sister helped her with the initial interpretation of the instructions, my participation was limited to the purchase of the small stamped metal bells which she embedded in the discarded nylon hose used to stuff each ball. At one time, shortly before the first Christmas, it was difficult to move around in our living room without tripping over a knitted ball. She made them in several sizes, from about two inches to six inches, and in all the colors of the rainbow, often suiting the color combinations to the season or holiday. Red and green were for Christmas; red, white, and blue for national holidays, and so on.

Following the period of the knitted balls she started a lengthy project of crocheting 192 multicolored squares which eventually would be crocheted together to form an afghan shawl. Betty had seen such an afghan shawl, recently completed, in the home of an admired neighbor and shortly thereafter had started to crochet one for herself. Handiwork in the form of knitting or crocheting has provided a mentally restful outlet for her naturally busy nature.

7

The Second Year

The daily routine of speech therapy continued to be the principal activity of Betty's life. Slowly the wheel of existence turned, with the radial spokes of social activity and the rim of household problems revolving around the hub of speech.

Stenographer's loose-leaf notebooks were used as work sheets for the language lessons and Betty carried them back and forth between home and the hospital. They became filled so rapidly that she soon decided to buy a large, black leatherlike bag in which to carry all the notebooks, voice tapes, glasses, gloves, etc. She selected it for its ample capacity for meeting her needs and it was amazing the number of items that got tucked away in that bag. Whenever Betty had misplaced or lost something of a personal nature, which was rather frequently, we always looked in the large black bag first.

The variety of subjects which came cascading helter-skelter out of the pages of the notebook each week seemed to be a mishmash of details and unrelated events, but when they were examined in perspective there was a common thread of affinity running through all of them. I recognized this common thread to be relevance to everyday living. Any subject or event which would excite the interest of Betty the woman, Betty the housewife, Betty the mother and grandmother, Betty the librarian, Betty the club woman, Betty the citizen of the USA—be it an astronaut's first flight into space, or the arrival of a new grandchild, the cost of drycleaning, or a national election—that subject or happening eventually appeared in the notebook. And the time of its appearance was always in the period of maximum interest for Betty.

A typical example of the involvement of personal affairs was the annual luncheon meeting of the Study Club at which the past presidents were honored. Betty attended this meeting, the first for her since the stroke, but only after several weeks of inner struggle and after finally finding the courage to take this important step. She compromised by not going for the luncheon, but attending only the meeting afterward. A few days later Miss Simonson wrote the following question in the notebook: "What happened at the Study Club May 5?"

Betty's answer, written in pencil underneath the question is reproduced here:

> The Study Club at the Library Cultural Center Wednesday May 5. I did not go the lunch. I had coffee. The President order. Minutes. Past Presidents stand up. Member clap. Past President had orchid. (me). Betty Bryant new President next year. Many friends talk to me. Mr. Hoffmeier (Hudson driver) was mystery guest. (Laugh!) Betty brought me flowers (daisy) from table.

The wedding in the spring of the second year was another of the topical events which received its share of attention in the daily language lessons. Most women are thrilled by the beauty and sentiment associated with a church wedding, and this thrill is even more intense when a daughter is a member of the wedding party. So Miss Simonson took advantage of this occasion to spread it over several language lessons.

For one of the lessons prior to the wedding Betty filled in the final words of these unfinished sentences written in the notebook:

Miss Simonson	Betty
The wedding:	
The bride's name is	Judy Elain Barkdull
The groom's name is	Douglas Franklin Westerkamp
The bridesmaids are	Margie Knox
The wedding will be at	Franklin Community Church
The reception will be at	church, and Douglas Westerkamp father house
The wedding will be on	May 8
at	7:30 P.M.
Margie will wear	pink dress, pink hat, pink shoes, white gloves, and flowers
Mrs. David Knox will wear	blue dress, blue hat (spider), black shoes, white gloves, black purse, and mink stole (?)
The newlyweds will live	at Ann Arbor

On another day Miss Simonson wrote three words: wedding, Judy, Saturday, and asked Betty to make up a sentence using them. Betty wrote, "I went Judy wedding on Saturday at church."

Later, following the wedding, Miss Simonson wrote in the notebook, "Tell about the wedding." Betty wrote as follows:

> The church is white and pew beige inside. The flowers were in two vases on the altar with candles. We sat left side. The organ is playing and minster came out. The girls are walking to the altar. The dress are pink and pretty. The bride wear white dress, veil, flowers and train. Margie was maid of honor and pretty. I went to reception lines—then punch and cake.

Evident here is some difficulty with verbs, but an improving vocabulary. In these examples, where composition was required, there were some words which she could say but could not visualize or spell. I would help her with the writing of these words so she could complete the sentence and get on with the composition. Once the word was written for her she would exclaim, "Oh, yes!" and her face would light up with recognition. Occasionally I would suggest a missing verb if its omission left the sentence bare or ambiguous. I had to fight the urge to supply all the missing words and to correct each little detail of composition. My role was secondary to the speech therapist, and I recognized that the composition should reveal to her the deficiencies which needed attention, as well as the breakthroughs in progress when they occurred.

The ability to pronounce a word does not mean, necessarily, that there is capability to write the word. This is probably rudimentary to the person trained in working with aphasics, but I had to learn to be patient when she could speak a word but could not spell or write it. Sometimes her effort to spell a word produced another word not even closely related to the first, for example, *every* might be written *want*. Perhaps the word *want* had some connection with the thought to be expressed later in her sentence.

As I thought more about it, it became clear that speech is related to the sound that is created by the voice and heard by the ears. No visualizing of the corresponding written word is required. Only the sound is important. On the contrary, to write a word or sentence requires first the visualizing of the letters or words in proper sequence. Most of us are not conscious of this thought process because writing and speaking have become such a strong habit. But for the aphasic, who has lost this process, a great deal of mental effort goes into the construction of even the simplest sentence.

Reading, too, is easier than writing because no creative effort is required, as in composition. The visualizing has been done by the writer and the reader needs only to register and interpret. But it was difficult for me to know how much Betty comprehended in reading, since she was not able to communicate this to me accurately. As she increased her ability to speak, I would ask questions about what she had been reading in such a way that she could give a meaningful reply. By this method I learned that her reading comprehension was fairly good. I could judge this also by noticing what she would pick up and read voluntarily. Her choice was always a news item or an article of a pragmatic nature—usually in a woman's magazine or *Reader's Digest*. Never did she read articles of an abstract nature which involved the imaginative thought process. Perhaps her reading comprehension could be best expressed by her own response to my question about her capability: "maybe one-half."

From time to time she would be emotionally overcome by extreme depression. There seemed to be no predictable regularity to the occurrence of these low points of morale. Sometimes they were triggered by a discernible stimulus, yet at other times the same stimulus would have no depressing effect. A real or imagined personal slight, a failure to write a word correctly when trying desperately to correspond, a sudden realization of exclusion from conversational gatherings; these were the types of stimuli which sometimes provoked depression. One day I discovered her sitting quietly on the sofa with tears streaming down her cheeks. After supplying a handkerchief I tried to find out what was disturbing her or what might have happened. With some reluctance and a great deal of hesitation she finally made it clear that she had been out walking and some older children had made fun of her speech and laughed at her.

These periods of depression were relatively short in duration—a matter of minutes or a few hours rather than days—and were almost always characterized by outbursts of "Why? Why?"—implying why did it happen, meaning the stroke, or why did it have to be me; or "Died! Died!"—meaning I wish I were dead or I wish I had died at the time of the stroke. In some of the more extreme seizures, which were very few, she would imply a desire for suicide by saying, "Dead! Dead! I will!"

At first I felt woefully inadequate in the face of these outbursts. Her feeling of depression would transfer to me and this tended to throttle my ability to help her throw off her emotional dejection. Gradually, as I experienced more of her valleys of despair, I could see what I had to do both for her and for me. I would remind her of people much more seriously afflicted—the blind, the paralyzed, and the deaf. She and I had much to be thankful for. She could see and enjoy beauty; she could walk; she could drive her car; she could see and hear her grandchildren, and do things with them and for them. We had many blessings that could fill our lives with happiness. I attempted to turn her thinking around toward the positive and brighter side of life and away from the problems of her handicap. Most of the time she would come out of it, finally smile with me, and return to being her normal cheerful and confident self.

Other times I tried to show her that achieving her goal of regaining speech and communication could be bigger than both of us. Her life could well be an inspiration to others similarly silenced at the peak of an active life. We had no way of knowing who, among our friends, acquaintances, or even children, might be similarly struck down in the future. And they would remember Betty and take heart, for if she could overcome this speech handicap and learn to live happily and constructively, so could they. Perhaps this was the answer to her oft-repeated cry of "Why? Why?"

Our housekeeper gave willingly of her time to Betty in working with her on the lessons, but it became increasingly apparent that her help was losing some of its effectiveness. Betty would try to describe the problem to me in private but was unable to communicate precisely what was bothering her. No household can be maintained by two women without occasional differences, especially when one is not a member of the family. Betty and Berniece did have their differences, and both tried to understand and to accommodate. But this problem was related to the speech lessons rather than to housekeeping, and I concluded that it had something to do with the ultrasensitivity of the aphasic.

It is likely that Betty's sensitivity and a possible subconscious display of impatience on the part of Berniece during a practice session led Betty to the erroneous conclusion that Berniece was not very understanding. I too have seen this sensitivity to a serious and supposedly helpful remark on my part result in a rejoinder from her, "Smiling please, smiling!" So it was not surprising that she would occasionally misconstrue some of Berniece's words as signs of impatience.

Betty had suggested to me privately that it might help if Berniece could talk with Miss Simonson about how she could be of more help at home. This seemed like a constructive suggestion. Accordingly I discussed the problem with Miss Simonson and she welcomed the opportunity to talk with Berniece if I would arrange for her to be the driver one day. Following this visit there was a noticeable improvement in their periods of working together, and the impending crisis faded away. We shall always be grateful to Berniece for generously and cheerfully performing a difficult but very necessary function in this period of our lives.

In June of the second year our youngest daughter, Margaret, received her degree from Michigan State University, and we eagerly prepared to be in East Lansing on graduation day for a parent's luncheon and the formal exercises following. This event marked the end of the ten-year span of college education for our three children, so we were understandably enthusiastic about observing this milestone. However, the trip to East Lansing grew to be more than just a passenger ride for Betty. She was to drive her car alone on the freeway for the first time, and for a distance of eighty miles.

Daughters in college dormitories are natural pack rats, and over a period of four years manage to put in one room more worldly goods than can be transported with one trip of an average car, especially with three human occupants to boot. So Margaret asked if her mother could drive the second car to East Lansing on Saturday, and she would drive it home on Monday filled with the remainder of her paraphernalia. This was a challenge for Betty over and above the challenge of attending the luncheon and meeting Margaret's friends. She had not driven on a freeway since her stroke, and had purposely chosen to use only the multiple-lane city streets to and from the hospital. She had never liked the pressure of high speeds on the freeway.

We decided that I would drive the lead car and she would follow in view of the complications often encountered getting on and off a limited access freeway. When one is not familiar with the route, decisions must be made quickly after reading the directions on the overhead signs. I knew that such quick decisions were beyond her capability.

We got away as planned on Saturday morning and agreed that we would stay in the right-hand lane all the way, holding our speed at 50 miles per hour. I believe I had my eyes cocked to the rear view mirror on that trip almost as much as on the highway in front of me. Even at 50 miles per hour we encountered a few cars traveling slower, which we passed when traffic was light. We arrived in East Lansing on schedule and parked in the lot in front of the dormitory. As I opened the door of Betty's car she slumped over the steering wheel with a satisfied expression of relief and said, "I made it!"

Although the graduation exercises were an anticlimax after our drive, we enjoyed every minute of our visit and were thrilled at the inspiring words of Chief Justice of the United States, Earl Warren, as he spoke at the ceremony. We arrived home that night tired but happy and proud of both our daughter and her gritty mother.

The first summer following Betty's two strokes I took my vacation (what was left following the trip to Mexico) as usual in August during the hay fever season, but we stayed home. The second year in August we decided to spend a week at Watervale, a family resort in the dune country on Lake Michigan. We had been going there at the same time annually for fourteen years, and we were well acquainted with many of the guests who also returned at the same time year after year. This was a prime factor in our decision to return to Watervale, for Betty would feel comfortable with these people and would enjoy the change of scenery. Her sister and brother-in-law also vacationed there annually at the same time, and our daughter Janet and her family usually returned each year to Watervale.

So this was a real opportunity for Betty to face up to new situations in different, yet familiar, surroundings. It also provided a necessary respite from the nose-to-the-grindstone activity associated with speech therapy. I, too, welcomed the opportunity to get away from our repetitive routine. All was not beer and skittles, however, for Betty soon selected picture post cards to send to friends. This meant about an hour or two each morning devoted to addressing cards and composing personal notes. Whenever possible, the same note was used over again on many cards.

Betty adapted very well to the new surroundings, went hiking with me along the beautiful Lake Michigan beach, visited our old friend Gwen Frostic in her new studio nearby on the Betsie River, and attended all the predinner parties with our friends of many years. Watervale was another speech laboratory where Betty put into practice all the improvement in speech and communication that she had made in her first year. She participated enthusiastically in a card game called "99," which involved card recognition, addition and subtraction, as well as speech; a game suited admirably to the carefree atmosphere of vacations. With patience on the part of the friendly players, Betty could enjoy the sociability and competition of the game. Most of all, Betty took great, unspoken satisfaction in her acceptance as a player by her friends.

The vacation was soon ended and we were back to the language lessons. It became more and more apparent to me that some of the most difficult words to define are little words such as the articles, *a, an,* and *the;* the interrogating words such as *who, what, why, where, when,* and *how;* the small adverbs such as *then, so, also, now,* and *as;* and many of the conjunctions and prepositions such as *and, if, but, to, of, from, in, on, at,* etc. We who are not teachers tend to forget how many of these little words there are in our language, and how very necessary and important they are to composition and communication.

It is small wonder that the aphasic has so much difficulty recovering the ability to use these little words properly. They do not represent anything that can be seen, touched, heard or sensed in any way; and, as Miss Simonson liked to put it, "They have no drama!" The dramatic words, the picturesque words, are the ones which are easiest to relearn and to adorn with meaning. Words such as *horse, water, flower, orange,* and *ice cream* come alive for the aphasic, especially when coupled with a picture.

This difficulty with the so-frequently used simple words is frustrating to a person working with the aphasic. I learned to be patient with Betty when she would write *if* instead of *from, the* instead of *to,* and many other such errors. Gradually I came to understand that improvement in this phase of language would take a lot of effort and a long time. Miss Simonson frequently introduced practice word combinations embracing articles, prepositions, and adverbs in the daily lesson. The following is typical:

Miss Simonson wrote	*Betty wrote*
Finish:	
Come to	the party
	the school
Go in	the store
	the dining room
Eat on	the table
	the patio
Comb with	the blue comb
	the hair comb
Put in	the salt
	the flour, egg, and butter
He sat on	the chair
	the sofa

This lesson proved to be a drill using the article, *the,* as well as practice using some prepositions. It would appear that the drab little words, of which we have so many, can only be learned by repeating them over and over again in their proper association with other words which provide meaning. The little words are never used alone. Only when combined with other words do they perform their function of tying the stark language elements into a living and meaningful thought expression.

I became aware of the formidable aspects of the little words about the time, in the fall of 1965, when we decided it would be fun to take Miss Simonson to dinner with us and become better acquainted with her after-hours personality. Betty's younger sister and her husband also agreed to join the festive little party at a popular eastside dining spot. And to top it off, Miss Simonson asked us to her apartment first for "Seven-up." To provide Betty with an active and conversational role at dinner I hurriedly prepared in advance a few little appropriate limericks for her to read. I had hoped that she might be able to memorize one, but this proved to be too much for her. The evening was a great success in spite of my extreme embarrassment when I, the practicing mechanical engineer, the one who knows all about cars, was unable to start my car as we left Miss Simonson's apartment for the restaurant. With the help of a taxi we overcame my deficiency of engineering talent. Betty was able to read some of the rapidly penned poems, which did provide some colorful participation for her. Although obviously amateur, they were all related to her aphasia. The first one went:

> To a lovely lady named Jo
> I was sent to when I was laid low.

She told me I could if only I would,
And words from my lips do now flow.

In rapid succession the other five were read aloud:

An aphasic needs help with her words,
And working alone's for the birds;
But to say the name Simonson before the work's begun
Seems just a little absurd.

Who, What, and *Why* are not easy
How, Have, and *Has* keep me busy
But the hardest of all are words very small
It, Is, and *I* make me dizzy.

Putting words in a sentence is rough
A noun and a verb's not enough
I don't understand the constant demand
For adjectives, adverbs, and fluff.

Reading aloud can be fun
The words that I miss almost none
I love to anticipate a big word before it's late
Usually before it has come.

Shakespeare, mathematics, umbrella,
Psychology, library, too
Are easier to say, if I had my way,
Than *no, the, on, in, it,* and *to.*

One of the highlights of the evening was Miss Simonson's expressed surprise at Betty's composure in a conversational group and especially her ability to understand conversation directed to her when others were talking in a noisy room. This ability to filter out conversation, so difficult for aphasics, was an accomplishment that Miss Simonson had not expected. I wondered if Betty's willingness to expose herself socially by dining out and going places generally, might have been a contributing factor to the progress.

Games that are not too complicated or sophisticated have provided a pleasant and relaxing pastime for both of us, although Betty would seldom agree to playing a game until her speech lesson was completed to her satisfaction. Games such as bridge or poker, requiring memory for what has been said by the other players, or requiring the use of deductive reasoning, are not for the aphasic. The rules of bridge and poker are relatively long and involved and a nimble mind is necessary just to be able to maintain a hand, to say nothing of achieving success.

We found pleasure in playing rummy as long as we played only the simple form and stayed away from the more complicated scoring procedures of gin rummy. Betty had good recall of the two possibilities for scoring—accumulating sequential runs and duplicating numerical values—and would beat me often enough to keep her interested.

Another game we played less frequently was cribbage, an ideal pastime for two people that we had enjoyed prior to her illness. She was not so successful at mastering the variety of scoring situations which make this such an attractive game, yet she tended to rise to the challenge. With help from me she was able to keep the game moving, but the result was something less than a contest. However, it did provide a painless way for her to practice adding numbers.

Scrabble was the game that we enjoyed most, and played most often. Curiously, this was the one game that was closely related to the language therapy program, yet Betty considered it recreation. I was amazed at how well she could construct the words, occasionally coming up with nouns she had not used before, or which had not appeared in her lessons. She was not able to pronounce some of the words, yet she recognized that the combination of letters was a familiar one and had meaning for her.

It occurred to me that Scrabble, or some off-shoot of Scrabble embracing individual letters, might be useful as a therapeutic procedure in specific aphasia cases. Undoubtedly, word games have been carefully studied and evaluated by people engaged in speech research. I was greatly impressed by how completely absorbed Betty would become searching for the proper word, and with what a feeling of elation she would announce her success. Understandably, she did not pay much attention to the double and triple word locations where the individual score would be greatly enhanced. She was happy if she could produce a word on the board, regardless of the score. And when she tired, that was the end of the game. She knew the limit of her capability. Many times I have observed this sudden onset of fatigue, and learned to heed it promptly.

Several years before Betty's illness I had formed the habit of walking at night, winter and summer, weather permitting. I would walk briskly for about a mile, and I found that my physical condition benefited from this mild exercise. It also served as a period of quiet contemplation for mulling over the problems that confronted me daily in my work. On those occasions when Betty would join me, both benefits obviously were diminished. Following her stroke, however, she became quite insistent about making the evening walk a part of her daily regimen. It was difficult at first for me to understand why she rejected my suggestion that she walk in the daytime. She would exhibit a shrinking posture of fear and repeat the words, "I can't!" It became clear that she would not risk a chance meeting with an acquaintance on the street, and thereby expose her speech handicap.

Even at night, while walking with me in the early days of her aphasia, Betty would direct our steps across the street if someone was approaching us. She soon overcame this extreme sensitivity, but even today she will not walk very often in the daylight. This continuing sensitivity seems inconsistent with her willingness to shop in the supermarket and department stores.

Walking at night was more than fresh air and exercise for her. It was an occasion for working on her speech. She would ask me to talk to her while walking, and would attempt to repeat some of my words. I would comment on the weather and try to have her repeat "It is cold," or "It is cloudy," or "It is dark." The subjects we used in our simple conversation were taken mostly from our visible surroundings, nature's sky, trees, grass, or man-created houses, streets, cars, etc. Sometimes an important happening of the day, such as the launching of an astronaut into space, would be powerful enough to drive our thoughts and rudimentary conversation beyond the horizon of our surroundings.

It occurred to me that one of the advantages of this kind of speech therapy is the unending supply of stimuli that are encountered while walking, and they are all either visual or auditory. The aphasic person, if not lacking in imagination, has difficulty expressing thoughts or words which are products of the imagination. But he readily responds to a visual stimulus or to

a sound stimulus. A crack of thunder, followed by saying the word "thunder," is a good illustration of using
an external stimulus in speech therapy. Walking outside
presents a continuous supply of fresh stimuli. When the
weather was bad we would sit in the living room and
Betty would ask me to quiz her by pointing to objects
in the room. She would repeat the name of the object,
if known to her, but we soon ran out of available objects and had to move into another room.

It was in the spring of 1965, about one year after the
first stroke, that Betty evidenced an interest in seeing a
movie. Not just any movie, but a particular movie she
had seen advertised in the newspaper. "Mary Poppins"
conjured up pleasant memories of a little girl's book;
and with Julie Andrews as the vocal star it was not surprising that Betty should show an enthusiasm for seeing this picture. I could not be certain how well she
would follow the dialogue, but I was sure that the music would hold her interest. As it turned out, she enjoyed every minute of the evening. Her understanding
of the dialogue, with the help of the pictorial presentation, was excellent, and she was stimulated to talk
about the evening's entertainment, in her limited way,
for some time.

This experience was followed, a few months later, by
"My Fair Lady"; and later that year we attended another Julie Andrews triumph, "The Sound of Music."
As far as Betty was concerned "The Sound of Music"
was the epitome of entertainment and enjoyment. She
loved the light music, and the plot was straightforward
enough for her to follow in spite of her aphasia. We can
confidently recommend the light musical type of mo-

tion picture as good entertainment for the aphasic, especially in the early stages of recovery.

Later, at her urging, we attended a showing of "Dr. Zhivago" because Betty had seen so much favorable publicity in the news media in the form of reviews. In spite of the length of this picture and its somber sophistication she willingly stayed to the end, and enjoyed it for the most part. Not surprisingly her subsequent questions confirmed my suspicion that there were certain passages in this picture that moved too swiftly, or were too subtle, for her to comprehend completely.

Since then we have seen "Thoroughly Modern Millie," "Camelot," "The Graduate," "Guess Who's Coming to Dinner," and "Hawaii." The inclusion of the last three, not one of which is musically oriented, is a measure of Betty's improvement in word and thought understanding. As might be expected, the least enjoyed was "The Graduate," but more because of the generation gap in moral values than because of any basic lack of comprehension.

Word recall for the aphasic individual is very unpredictable, but when it happens it can be startling to a companion, and sometimes to the afflicted person. I have witnessed it many times and wondered how the word signal managed to get through the brain barrier. I have also pondered over the wonderful word storage facility of the brain, and what happens to this facility when stroke damage takes place. Is it functionally intact? Is the damage limited to the switching network that releases words to the transmitting circuit? Are the words only locked up, waiting for the development of a new channel for their release? The gradual reappearance of more and more of the "lost" words would tend to strengthen this idea.

I recall vividly the circumstances related to a dramatic demonstration of this unexpected word recall late in the second year after Betty's strokes. We had retired about ten o'clock that evening and were lying quietly in bed, Betty, looking at a woman's magazine and I, reading a book. Berniece had returned to her home for the weekend, so there was no one else in the house. Suddenly there was a noise that startled both of us. It seemed to originate from inside the house and it sounded like a person's footstep. Betty put down her magazine and looked at me questioningly. I got up immediately and made a tour of the house from the second floor to the basement, turning on the lights as I went. After finding nothing unusual, and deciding that the noise had probably originated outside the house, I returned upstairs to the bedroom and told Betty of my findings and my conclusion. As I got into bed, she said quite clearly, "Spooky!" Not believing what I heard I said, "What did you say?" She repeated, but louder this time, "Spooky!"

I am certain that the word had never appeared in any of her speech lessons, and I am also sure that we had had no previous occasion, since her stroke, to use that word. But there it was, suddenly and dramatically released from its long imprisonment.

8

Group Therapy

The announcement that our speech therapist was leaving Henry Ford Hospital the first of December to take a supervisory position in the speech clinic at the University of Michigan was a disturbing blow to the stability of our lives. We had become accustomed to a routine completely devoted to Betty's improvement, and when December came and there was no replacement in sight for Miss Simonson at Ford Hospital, the future appeared bleak and lacking in fulfillment. Betty was more resolutely motivated than ever toward driving herself to the limit to recover her speech, but it would take more than motivation and drive. It would again require the direction and inspiration of one skilled and experienced in the art of speech rehabilitation.

In the early days of Betty's struggle we had given some consideration to a resident class in group therapy for aphasics at the University of Michigan in Ann Arbor. It had been my judgment at that time that Betty would progress more rapidly if she could live and study in the familiar and comfortable surroundings of her own home. Now, once more, we gave consideration to looking at the group therapy program in Ann Arbor, but again decided against it. We continued to rationalize that she would improve faster in her own home.

So we put out feelers for finding a speech therapist nearby who would either see Betty on a regular schedule in the office, or who would, hopefully, come to our home for the lesson. Of the two practitioners who were brought to our attention we selected a young lady who was known to a respected friend of Betty's. This young lady was a graduate speech major and was teaching speech to retarded children in the public schools. Her schedule permitted coming to our house two afternoons a week for one-hour sessions. She was a capable teacher, personable, and devoted to her professional work, and Betty was quite happy with the arrangement. She buckled down to her new routine after the winter holidays, and now she had more time for other activities since there was no time lost driving to the speech lesson.

The following spring, at Miss Simonson's urging, we drove to Ann Arbor one day to visit the class in group therapy at the University of Michigan. This day was a memorable one for both of us, more especially for me because it brought home so dramatically the beneficial impact of group activity.

We arrived at the clinic at midmorning coffee hour and all the patients were in the commons room for conversation and informal socializing. One of the patients was pouring and asked, with one word and a gesture, if we would like coffee. Of course we would. Another passed cookies, and Miss Simonson introduced us to each of the patients as well as to members of the staff who also were enjoying this coffee break with the patients. I had the unmistakable impression that all of these people, handicapped as they were and some with partial paralysis, were happy in each other's company and in their common endeavor.

I conversed with two of the men, each of whom had spent about a year at the speech clinic following strokes. One was a lawyer of some importance and the other was a top sales executive with a division of General Motors. They talked with some hesitation but their vocabulary was adequate and they communicated quite well with me. Both had praise for the effectiveness of group therapy as it was practiced at the university. Obviously they recognized that they would not be able to carry on in their responsible positions without the improvement they were making in speech.

The group was composed of both men and women and they represented a wide range of economic and cultural backgrounds. I could sense that Betty would be comfortable in a group such as this. After we made a complete tour of the facilities, including the dormitory and dining room, and after viewing and listening to some of the speech classes from behind one-way windows, Miss Simonson suggested that Betty should plan on spending another day at the clinic in the near future, being tested and appraised for her acceptability into the speech-rehabilitation program. I accepted tentatively pending further discussion with Betty. I had learned that aphasics take a great deal of time in making decisions. Their lack of retention of immediate thoughts does not permit the rapid weighing of alternatives, the juggling of ideas back and forth, that we are accustomed to doing so effortlessly in decision making. If pressed for a quick decision the aphasic will usually choose the status quo.

Later when we were alone at home I suggested that Betty need not make up her mind immediately about joining the speech class in Ann Arbor. She could take the qualification tests without being committed to the program. After all, she might be rejected for some reason. If they accepted her, we could then decide about her taking the group instruction. We would have plenty of time to prepare for the move to Ann Arbor since the next session for which she would be eligible would not start until after the July fourth holiday.

As time went on I spelled out the answers to some of the questions that I knew she would have. I was convinced that the right decision was for her to enroll in the University of Michigan speech clinic, but I had to convince her. So I focused her attention on all the favorable aspects. I reminded her that she would see Josephine Simonson every day, so she would not be entirely among strangers. I told her I would bring her home every Friday night and return her to Ann Arbor Sunday evenings. That way, she would be away from home only five days each week. Berniece would take care of our home, do the washing and ironing, and prepare my meals, so she need not be concerned about my welfare while she was away. I would call her on the telephone as often as she wished and she could call me any evening. The clincher turned out to be the fortunate fact that both of our married children lived in Ann Arbor and she would be able to visit her grandchildren more often.

When we went to Ann Arbor to take the evaluation tests Betty already had decided that she wanted to join the class in group therapy. She was accepted in May as being capable of meeting the rigorous requirements of the speech program, and so we enrolled her in the speech class in July.

At the start of each five-week term at the University of Michigan Speech Clinic, members of the immediate family are invited and urged to join the patient at a get-acquainted tea with members of the staff; this is scheduled for the Sunday afternoon preceding the opening day of instruction. Our group meeting proceeded quite informally, following an introduction of the patients and members of the staff, and a presentation of the history of the clinic, its objectives and accomplishments. It was interesting to learn that the patients came from many distant states as well as from Michigan.

We were particularly buoyed by an interview with two former patients conducted by Miss Simonson before the assembled families. Both were men from the business world, one a certified public accountant and the other a sales executive of a large automotive company. They had "graduated" from the speech clinic and returned to a semiactive life. Although their conversation was slower and more painstaking than that of a normal person, they both displayed a remarkable recovery that was heartening to us. Both stressed that the use of the telephone presents a formidable problem to the aphasic, a difficulty compounded by not being able to see the other party's facial expressions and hand and body gestures. Truly, the telephone can be a fearful monster to the aphasic.

The CPA had retired from his previous position as a result of his stroke, but felt that he might still be able to handle some income tax business for small firms or individuals on a part-time basis. He said it had taken him several days to force himself to make the first telephone call. He was in a nervous sweat and his hand shook as he dialed the number, hoping that the line would be busy. Fortunately, the party answered and as soon as he started to talk his confidence returned. He knew from that first telephone conversation that he now was capable of doing this kind of work, and has continued to compute income tax returns on a part-time basis.

Common to both men was the problem of their ability to communicate diminishing as they became tired. A great deal of effort is expended by the aphasic in speech and writing, so by the time afternoon rolls around they have pretty well "had it" for that day.

I had some misgivings about leaving Betty that first time with a group of strangers, but when I called for her the following Friday evening she was bubbling with enthusiasm about the program, arduous as it was. As we departed through a lounge where many of the patients were watching television, Betty said goodbye to each one until Monday. I, too, started to get acquainted with the patients and felt sorry for those who were facing a dismal institutional weekend away from home. The ones who were ambulatory, however, were free to come and go, and could go out for meals or for a walk in the fresh air if they wanted a change.

Betty's day at the clinic started at 6:30 A.M. Since she had an alarm clock which I had set for her, she volunteered to awaken the other two ladies in adjacent rooms. Breakfast in the dining room was at 7 A.M. Her speech therapy schedule was typical and started at 8 A.M. with a class in group therapy with two other patients. From 9 A.M. to 10 A.M. was an open hour. Sometimes this open period would be used for research work by staff or doctoral candidates, inasmuch as Betty had volunteered to assist as a patient in this work.

The coffee hour was from 10 A.M. to 11 A.M. in the commons room; but Betty's name for this room was "the coffee shop," and this name was soon picked up and used by some of the others. All patients were expected to attend the social hour in this room as it was considered an important aspect of the therapy program.

Another session in speech therapy, this time individual instruction rather than group, was scheduled from 11 A.M. to 12 noon and was followed by the lunch hour when all the patients assembled in the dining room. Even the dining periods did not escape the overtones of speech therapy, and some of the staff members were always present to stimulate conversation and try to draw all of the patients into an exchange of ideas.

From 1 P.M. to 2 P.M. she had another class in group therapy with three other patients. Her last class, a group activity with two others, was from 2 P.M. to 3 P.M. The balance of the afternoon, as well as the evening, was for rest or study in the dormitory rooms. For the most part the patients devoted the time to their speech and writing assignments, usually working in pairs or in groups. Miss Simonson informed me that they worked like "dogs" on these assignments trying to improve themselves and in the evening they were utterly exhausted.

Betty attended four successive five-week programs at the Aphasia Division of the University of Michigan Speech Clinic, extending over the period from July to the end of the following February. A written evaluation of her progress was provided about the middle of each program. I was invited to attend the sessions on the final day of each program as an observer behind one-way glass windows. Following the sessions I took advantage of the opportunity to confer with each of the clinicians regarding her progress.

Although she made significant advances in all aspects of communication—listening, speaking, reading, and writing—I believe Betty's greatest improvement was in self-confidence and socializing. An illustration of this is shown in part of the evaluation written by the senior clinician during the last program in February:

> There is one other aspect of communication which Miss Bell worked on last semester and that I plan to emphasize during these last two weeks—that of self-confidence. As you may know, Mrs. Knox went by herself to University Hospital for her appointment in Ophthalmology. She did not know exactly where to go, but by asking people she found her own way and talked with the doctor by herself. I feel that this was a great step forward in independence, and I hope to provide more opportunities for her to "make her own way" before she leaves. She can do it if she's willing to try!
>
> Mrs. Knox has continued to act as our hostess in coffee hour, making and serving tea, passing cookies, and generally helping others to feel comfortable. Her graciousness will be sorely missed when she leaves.

I was impressed with the beneficial aspects of group therapy for aphasics. I witnessed the stimulating effect on each of the patients in a group session—the giving and taking that went on among them. When one didn't know the answer—or couldn't say it—another would provide it. They offered and received criticism from one to another. But they also were free with their praise for a good performance. They understood each other, for they had a common problem. The mental cross-stimulation between members of such a handicapped group is marvelous to observe.

After pondering over the impact of group therapy in communications, as opposed to individual therapy, I submit the following as possible contributing factors to personal progress:

(1) Minimizing the feeling of isolation. "I am not the only one with this problem."

(2) Providing the motivation of competition. "If he can do it, I can do it better."

(3) Satisfying the gregarious urge. The human being is naturally gregarious. A group of people having the same problem and goal will band together quickly and enthusiastically.

(4) Satifying the need for praise. Praise from a fellow aphasic can be more poignant than praise from the teacher.

(5) Satifying the need for understanding. The aphasic is never sure of the teacher's complete understanding of what it means to be an aphasic. This understanding can not be conveyed, for obvious reasons, but he knows that a fellow-aphasic understands him completely.

(6) With mutual understanding comes a diminishing of fear. Diminishing of fear promotes self-confidence, which in turn overcomes the tendency for withdrawal.

Living with aphasics, which meant eating together, studying together, and socializing in general, contributed greatly to the progress Betty made. She was participating in a program with people again. She was imbued with a desire to help others, to express herself more openly—even if haltingly—to excel when possible and to converse more and more. She came to be known as "the Elsa Maxwell of the Speech Clinic" because of her desire and ability to carry out the role of the hostess.

Almost daily some event was found to be a cause for celebration, and this promoted the interchange of speech in a friendly social atmosphere. Someone on the staff would have a birthday (real or imagined), one of the patients would have a birthday, a new grandchild would be born (it happened to Betty), a new satellite would be launched or another news event of national significance would occur, St. Valentine's Day, Ground Hog Day, or Columbus Day, almost anything having some meaning to the group was used as an excuse for celebration and discussion. Sometimes a cookout was arranged for variety and to give the members of the group participation in meal preparation and serving, as well as to become better acquainted with the staff. I recall one occasion when Betty wrote all of the personal invitations to a birthday celebration for one of the leading members of the staff—and this was no small task for an aphasic.

Her weekends at home started when I would arrive in Ann Arbor Friday afternoon in time to take her out to dinner, usually at one of the University dining rooms. She enjoyed the change in atmosphere of getting home, and by Sunday afternoon she would have her bag packed with freshly laundered clothes and be ready to return. Since Berniece left for her home on Friday, we would be alone for the weekend, and there was ample opportunity to talk about the happenings of the past week at the speech clinic. Once I was prevented from driving the forty miles to Ann Arbor by a devastating snow storm. When I called Betty on the telephone she understood my dilemma. The next morning our son-in-law drove her home. She had called her daughter on the phone, as she was accustomed to doing frequently now, to tell her that she was staying in Ann Arbor because of the storm. Betty was becoming quite communicative in her use of the telephone.

Her final term at the speech clinic was over at the end of February and Betty had a little difficulty understanding why she was not going back for further help. The explanation that the program at Ann Arbor had accomplished all that could be accomplished for her, and that from now on she would continue to improve by practice at home did not completely satisfy her overwhelming desire for perfection. A vacation that we spent in Florida during the month of March helped her to make the transition.

Did I make the wrong decision by not enrolling Betty at the University of Michigan Speech Clinic immediately following her first or even her second stroke? Would group therapy have made that much difference in her recovery? I can never know the answer to that question.

Post Therapy—
What Now?

The closing of the period of formal speech therapy need not and should not be considered the end of all effort at speech improvement. Betty was still highly motivated and continued to apply herself, with some help from me, to reading assignments suggested by the speech clinician in Ann Arbor.

News For You is a weekly newspaper consisting of two folded pages, published by Laubach Literary, Inc. for adults who have a deficiency in vocabulary. It is published in two editions, A edition being an easier version than B edition. Betty and the other patients had used the A edition at the speech clinic in Ann Arbor, so I took out a subscription for Betty to read at home. However, as Betty gradually resumed her interest in our local newspaper her interest in *News For You* lagged. After one year I did not renew the subscription. She apparently looked upon *News For You,* perched on our news rack for all to see, as a symbol of her handicap. And it was evident that she had become quite proficient in reading and understanding at least some of the standard newspaper items.

She would call my attention to announcements of engagements or weddings of interest to us. And of course, she always read the obituaries and pointed out the references to friends or acquaintances. More recently she showed me a rather lengthy special news item that carried only one reference to the name of a neighbor who was assisting in a program for handicapped children. This name was buried in the middle of the article, so she must have read a considerable portion of it to come across the familiar name.

Another reading assignment that Betty worked on at the speech clinic was a simplified version of Hawthorne's *House of the Seven Gables*. Since she had not finished it by the end of her term we continued to sit down together frequently in the evening so she could read aloud from the book. At the end of each chapter we would make use of the reference questions as exercises for conversation and vocabulary drill. If she did not have the answer to a question, which was quite often, she would refer back to the text material and find the proper reference to give the answer.

Later, after my retirement, when we visited our youngest daughter who was now a hospital dietitian in Boston, we visited the House of the Seven Gables in Salem, Massachusetts. This was one of the high points of Betty's trip. She thrilled at seeing some of Hawthorne's descriptions come to life in the restored version of the famous house.

This paperback book was but one of a series of the American Classics published by Regents Publishing Company and has a vocabulary range of 750 words. I purchased two others suggested by Betty. They were *Portrait of A Lady* and *The Red Badge of Courage,* with a vocabulary range respectively of 2000 words and 2600 words. At Betty's insistence we started next on *The Red Badge of Courage,* with its formidable array of new multisyllable words. It has taken over a year to finish this book, but, in all fairness, we have not been as systematic in our devotion to reading aloud as we might have been. In retrospect it would have been more logical to select the books in the prescribed order of gradual increase of vocabulary range. For instance, *Moby Dick* has a range of 1000 words, the original 750 words used in "Seven Gables" with the addition of 250 new ones. The word range of the books increases from there to 1200, to 1400, to 1600, up to 2600.

We found reading aloud from these books quite helpful because it tended to satisfy Betty's urge to do something to improve herself. There were times, however, when an unusual number of new words would appear and she would express discouragement over the amount of help she needed from me for pronunciation. Too often we would wait until evening for this exercise, and her fatigue would contribute to a poor performance. I know now that difficult reading is best done by the aphasic earlier in the day. I also know that it can be a tedious lackluster session for the reading companion, for she has caught me several times with drooping or closed eyelids as she droned through the words. I would awaken with a start when she said, "Eyes! Eyes!" I was expected to correct her errors of pronunciation, or to supply the unmanageable word.

At the other extreme I was guilty many times of saying the word for her, before she had given up, before she was ready to accept help. Her irate outbursts let me know how important it was for her to do it herself. Sometimes, after Betty has said a word incorrectly, I have supplied the correct word without thinking to ask her to try again, for it is not always easy to know if she is ready to give up. "One and two! One and two!", she will snap, meaning that she always wants a second try before I intercede.

Working with Betty as she reads aloud has made me keenly aware that she often understands the meaning of the printed word but is unable to pronounce it. It is very evident from the following list of actual examples that she speaks a word very closely associated with the one she is attempting to say. Sometimes a second attempt will produce the correct word.

What was printed in the book:	*Betty's first attempt to say the word:*
stare	eyes
mechanical	engineer
brain	mind
relatives	family
flew	air
galloping	horsing
felt	left
taxi	cab
sergeant	colonel
oath, or swear	damn, damn
bullet	shot

She often laughs as she says such words for she knows they are not correct. She also knows that many are suitable as synonyms. Some of the words come out without thinking. The first flash that comes to her mind provides the impetus for a fast answer. The satisfaction of speed is worth the risk of an error.

Betty's spelling reveals some of the same shadings of error as her reading. For the most part, however, the written errors are limited to the little words and often reveal a tendency to shorten some of the longer words.

The word Betty wanted to write:	*The word she wrote:*
sausage	saugage
from	for
there	they
home	house
thine	thy
temptation	temption
affectionately	affectionaly
banana	bana

Awareness of her handicap is most acute for her when she is trying to converse. She refuses to be satisfied with less than her prestroke ability, even though friends as well as the doctors tell her how well she is doing and what a remarkable recovery she has made. "Not good. Not good!", she will say. (Repetition is common in her speech, and probably is a kind of crutch to fill in with more words.)

I am sure most of us in the same circumstances would assume the same attitude of not settling for less than normal conversational speech, for we would understand, as Betty does, that her social semi-isolation results from her inability to contribute in a completely normal manner to either individual or group conversation. This phenomenon of finding herself "left out" has been most difficult for her to accept, and the adjustment to this unfortunate facet of our new life probably will never be complete. Accommodation, perhaps; but acceptance, no. Friends and relatives have been very kind and thoughtful, and often go overboard to help fill in her decimated social calendar. She often takes the initiative in arranging social get-togethers, and this gives her solid satisfaction. I encourage her as much as possible. But the inevitable and, to me, understandable lulls in social activity depress her and lead to frequent repetition of the cry, "Why? Why?"

"Speak slowly. Slowly, please." Many times has she said this to me in order to understand more completely the meaning of what I have been saying. And when I speak slowly after the admonishment, her understanding is usually quite complete. Despite my long association with Betty throughout the long period of her speech deficiency, I still find myself lapsing into the normally rapid speech pattern to which most of us are accustomed. So it is not surprising, when we are conversing with friends, that a fully satisfying conversation is not always possible for her. In some situations when we are in a small group I have tried to set an example by adopting a slower tempo in my speech pattern. And if the friends are of long standing and she is at ease in their company she will often say "What? What?", or "Please, again" in an effort to have them repeat what was said. Most of the time this is enough to make the speaker aware that talking more slowly is necessary for good communication.

One of the more irritating actions on the part of an unthinking person is to direct an entire conversation to me, without once looking at Betty. I am conscious of this and, feeling self-conscious about it, I will look at Betty hoping that the other person will take the hint. On some occasions Betty has spoken out, and asked the person to talk to her. I sometimes wonder if any of my actions have tended to encourage leaving her out of the conversation. I hope not!

A cocktail party, of course, is quite a different conversational setting. She has apparently achieved a fairly high level of tolerance for the conglomerate of sounds that come cascading from all directions into her ears. The ability to filter out the immediate personal conversation from the confusing general noise is usually most difficult for the aphasic, but Betty seems to have partially achieved it. And it helps to locate her off to the side and out of the mainstream of cacophony.

Complete and clear-cut communication is difficult to achieve even among nonaphasic individuals, and this is true even among intellectuals whose conversation embraces the complexities of contemporary society. To the aphasic, however, the simple and familiar activities of everyday existence are difficult to communicate accurately. A typical example of this problem occurred one morning when Betty had a few skirts to go to the dry cleaner's. We were accustomed to taking our dry cleaning to one of our local businesses—which I shall call Jenny Smith—and already had several pieces of clothing there which could not be picked up until after 5 P.M. that day.

I said to Betty, "I will take your skirts to the cleaner's when I get the car washed this morning."

"No, you go to Jenny Smith and come back home today."

115

"Yes, I understand. But they will not have them cleaned today. Your skirts will not be ready until tomorrow. They will not do them in one day."

"Please! Please! You get the skirts today. You go to Jenny Smith today."

"Honey, I will take them today, as you wish. But I don't think they will have them ready tonight."

"No! No! No! Please honey, Jenny Smith today." She was so frustrated that she was bordering on tears. A few more minutes of this and it finally dawned upon me what she was trying to tell me. And it was so logical and simple. I had forgotten about the other items to be picked up, and she was suggesting that I take the skirts to Jenny Smith at 5 P.M. when I would be going to pick up the other items. Thus, I would be spared an extra trip.

This episode is typical of the occasional frustrating misunderstandings which stem from inadequate communication. If her first statement had been "No, you go to Jenny Smith and come back home *tonight*," I would likely have been reminded of the clothing that I was to pick up after 5 P.M. One must learn not to take literally what is said by the aphasic, for there may be a key word missing or misused. To pause before answering—like counting to ten—is not always easy, but may often be necessary.

Although the level of recovery Betty has made of the ability to speak, to read, to write, and to understand has been a satisfying and rewarding accomplishment, it still falls far short of what we would like to see her achieve. It is probably a rare occurrence when a person suddenly thrust into the depths of aphasia is able to climb all the way back to her former level of communication. In Betty's case the second jolt probably swept away any imminent possibility for complete recovery. We will keep trying, however, for the slow, steady improvement that faith and time may provide.

The following illustrations show Betty's ability to communicate; the intended meaning is usually clear and understandable, yet they portray the fine line between "getting by" and the accepted usage. For instance, she often will say "long" when she means "large" in describing an object. She uses the word "sad" for a great variety of unpleasant or unsatisfactory situations. When she says, "The music is sad," or "The television play is sad," she invariably means that it is objectionable, rather than melancholy. An oil painting is "sad" if it is modern enough to be confusing. "Shut the window" sometimes means to close the door, sometimes to draw the shade, and sometimes just what it says, to close the window. Substituting the word "open" for "shut" carries the same multiple possibilities. There are other words which fall into the same category, but these are typical.

She understandably creates and uses speech short cuts, sometimes in an ingenious way. We all use flowery adjectives to describe our opinion or rating of any and all objects and experiences, but not Betty. She has adopted a short cut that is quite descriptive and effective, as well as being widely applicable. When asked how she likes the food in a restaurant, she may reply, "B." That is all, just "B." This means that it is almost tops, but not quite. A "C" rating is pretty bad. The same system is used for movies, purchased items, perishable foods, television programs, art objects, etc. When asked how she feels, however, she usually says, "pretty good," "fine," or "sad." This likely indicates a trend toward more precise description as time goes on.

She sometimes, although rarely, uses a word that is completely wrong. These errors are probably associated with fatigue or lapse of memory. Most of us experience the latter as we grow older. She sometimes says the wrong day, for instance, saying Thursday when she means Friday. She may also say August when she really means to say October. Attempting to speak too rapidly also can lead to such errors. When corrected, she is likely to say, "That's what I said." Now that we have an air-conditioning system in the car, as well as a heater, she will ask for heat on a hot day when she means to ask for cool. The location of the control buttons or levers in the same area of the instrument panel probably contributes to this error.

"Nice to see you again, honey," is her customary conclusion to a telephone conversation. There is really nothing wrong with this statement, unless one is a purist and expects perfection. It is always understood by the listener, so it must convey the meaning intended. How wonderful to be capable of being understood again.

What I call crutch words are apt to creep into the aphasic's conversation and become part of his vocabulary. Betty uses the word "again" time after time as a sort of filler, and most of the time it does not change the meaning of what she is saying. "It is eleven o'clock. I will go to bed again." "We will go to the restaurant tonight again." In both of these examples the word "again" is superfluous, and is not intended to imply an additional happening. As noted previously, word repetition also is frequently used, but not necessarily for emphasis. It is my belief that repetition provides a sense of the rapid-fire conversation that once was so effortless; and it also tends to minimize the sound void while attempting to compose the next phrase.

Contrary to the emphasis here on some of Betty's deficiencies, I have not intended to minimize the slow but steady improvement she has made during the period following formal therapy. Her vocabulary has expanded, her confidence has increased, and there is every reason to expect that, with her dedication to achieving normalcy, she will continue to improve in all phases of communication.

Her triumph is one of the spirit as much as a victory over the vacuum in communication. Her speech is minimal, but adequate for simple conversation. Her understanding of the spoken word is fair. Her composition in writing leaves much to be desired. Yet she valiantly and resolutely embarks on social excursions. She shops in the supermarket and in department stores alone, and battles her way through the inevitable misunderstandings.

She initiates telephone calls and holds conversations. She visits new neighbors and exhibits her shortcomings to strangers unabashed. She attends women's club and church group meetings, although mostly to listen and rub elbows rather than to participate. She attends noisy cocktail parties and wedding receptions, maintaining her end of the conversation with a soft drink. Altogether, she is a stronger person for having won a thrilling victory over great odds. Perhaps this is one of the answers to her plaintive, "Why? Why?" And as for me, there is nothing more satisfying than to be on the side of the victor—to be a member of a winning team.

David Knox is the retired director of a large engineering company in Detroit, Michigan. He attended Wayne State University and received his B.S. from the Massachusetts Institute of Technology (1927). His numerous civic responsibilities have included a period serving as the Mayor of the City of Huntington Woods, Michigan (1948–50), as chairman of the Planning Commission of the City of Huntington Woods (1950–54), and as a member of the Board of Directors of the Macomb County Traffic Safety Commission.

The manuscript was edited by Sandra Yolles. The book was designed by Don Ross. The type face for the text in linotype Times Roman designed by Stanley Moriso in 1931; and the display face is Prisma.

The text is printed on S. D. Warren's Olde Style Antique. The book is bound in Interlaken's Arco Linen cloth over boards. Manufactured in the United States of America.